IS EVISTA® FOR YOU?

- Are you a postmenopausal woman?
- Do you have a family history of breast cancer?
- Are you concerned about osteoporosis?
- Are you concerned about heart disease?
- Are you reluctant to take estrogen because of concern about breast cancer?
- Have you talked to your doctor about Evista?

evista®

(raloxifene)

A MEDICAL DOCTOR ANSWERS ALL YOUR QUESTIONS ABOUT THE NEW F.D.A.—APPROVED "MIRACLE" DRUG FOR WOMEN

MARK STOLAR, M.D.
and GREG A. ANNUSSEK

A CMD PUBLISHING BOOK

WHOLE CARE

AN AVON BOOK

The ideas, procedures, and suggestions in this book are intended to supplement, not replace, the medical advice of a trained medical professional. All matters regarding your health require medical supervision. Consult your physician before adopting the suggestions in this book, as well as about any condition that may require diagnosis or medical attention. The authors and publisher disclaim any liability arising directly or indirectly from the use of this book.

Evista(TM) is a registered trademark of Eli Lilly and Company.

AVON BOOKS, INC.
1350 Avenue of the Americas
New York, New York 10019

Published by arrangement with CMD Publishing, a division of Current Medical Directions, Inc.
Library of Congress Catalog Card Number: 98-94879
ISBN: 0-380-80500-6
www.avonbooks.com/wholecare

First Wholecare Printing: July 1999

WHOLECARE TRADEMARK REG. U.S. PAT. OFF. AND IN OTHER COUNTRIES, MARCA REGISTRADA, HECHO EN U.S.A.

Printed in the U.S.A.

WCD 10 9 8 7 6 5 4 3 2 1

Contents

Introduction vii

Chapter 1 1
What Is Osteoporosis?

Chapter 2 21
Preventing Osteoporosis

Chapter 3 41
Living with Osteoporosis

Chapter 4 59
Evista and the New Selective Estrogen Receptor Modulators (SERMs)

Chapter 5 71
Using Evista to Help Prevent or Treat Osteoporosis

Chapter 6 87
How to Treat Your Menopausal Symptoms with Alternative and Other Therapies While Taking Evista

Chapter 7 109
Other Medications Used to Prevent or Treat Osteoporosis

Chapter 8 129
Diet, Exercise, and Alternative Therapies for Osteoporosis

Chapter 9 145
The Future of Evista and SERMs: Treating Heart Disease and Breast Cancer

Chapter 10 167
Take Charge of Your Health

Glossary 197

Index 207

Introduction

The decade of the 1990s has brought exciting new insights into the area of women's health. Doctors began to appreciate the devastating consequences of osteoporosis in the aging woman. Similarly, cardiovascular disease in women became an area of intense investigation. No longer willing to accept these illnesses as inevitable, patients and doctors alike began to work together to take a proactive approach toward disease prevention. Many new treatments for managing cholesterol levels came on the market in the early 1990s, and in the latter half of the decade, doctors were provided with new, powerful therapies for diagnosing and treating osteoporosis. This book examines a very promising new treatment in menopausal and postmenopausal women's health—Evista®. You will learn about this unique form of hormone replacement therapy and you will also be provided with a sound lifelong approach to risk reduction and health maintenance. By the time you finish this book, you will understand more about Evista, estrogen, and natural therapies that are designed to add productive, healthy years to the lives of every woman, and you will be able to make informed choices when you are discussing this important issue with your doctor.

1

What Is Osteoporosis?

Quick Fact: The cost of caring for osteoporosis-related fractures in the United States amounts to $14 billion a year ($38 million a day), and that figure is rising.

Mary, age forty, is an attorney. Recently her mother was diagnosed with osteoporosis after falling and injuring herself in her kitchen. She had to be placed in a nursing home because she could no longer care for herself. Mary was alarmed. She had heard that osteoporosis runs in families. At her last doctor's appointment she tried to discuss her risk for osteoporosis with her doctor but was told that as an active, healthy, premenopausal woman she need not concern herself with a problem that was years away. Unsatisfied, Mary sought advice from her gynecologist, who is also a woman in her early forties. Her gynecologist pointed out to Mary that although she was healthy, active, and years from menopause, she was indeed at high risk for osteoporosis. Busy with a career and a family, Mary had little time for any exercise except an occasional swim. Her diet, which often consisted of meals that she grabbed on the run, contained little calcium. The five cups of coffee she drank each day were bad for her bones, and the doctor noted that the ten years of smoking in her twenties may have thinned Mary's bones as well. Mary asked her doctor to order a bone density test, but she was told that such a test would be inappropriate at her age, as significant osteoporosis does not usually begin until approximately age fifty. But her doctor also advised her that getting regular weight-bearing exercise and more dietary calcium would go a long way to preventing the development of osteoporosis when she reaches her mother's age.

Osteoporosis has many faces. It strikes women from all walks of life and from every social and economic background. Whether you are a homemaker or a high-level executive, a couch potato or a weekend warrior on the athletic field, you may be at risk for this bone-weakening condition and not even realize it. More than 28 million Americans are affected by osteoporosis, according to the National Osteoporosis Foundation (NOF), which has characterized the condition as a "major public health threat." About 10 million people actually have osteoporosis, and another 18 million have weak bones that make them more likely to get it. Most of these people have at least one thing in common—they usually are women. One of the reasons that osteoporosis has reached almost epidemic proportions in the United States is that most women simply do not know the facts about keeping their bones healthy. Seventy-five percent of women between the ages of 45 and 75 have never even spoken to their doctors about osteoporosis, according to a recent Gallup survey, despite the fact that this age group is at high risk. It is no wonder that some women have misperceptions about the condition.

Myth: Osteoporosis is an unavoidable part of aging. Why should you worry about something that you cannot change?

Fact: Osteoporosis is a very preventable condition. It is not inevitable. Through proper diet, regular exercise, and the use of medications such as Evista® (raloxifene) when appropriate, you can keep your bones healthy for a lifetime.

Myth: You do not have to be concerned about osteoporosis if you are in good general health.

Fact: Osteoporosis should be a concern of every woman, regardless of overall health. It is virtually impossible to detect osteoporosis on your own. You may look and feel fine and still have bones that are weak and fragile. Only your doctor has the medical knowhow and high-tech equipment to check the health of your bones.

Myth: There is nothing that you can do about osteoporosis until you reach menopause.

Fact: The sooner you start fighting osteoporosis, the better. It is almost never too early to take practical steps to help prevent the condition.

Osteoporosis has enormous consequences on the health of American women. Because it is a silent disease—meaning that it does not cause symptoms early on—most women are unaware that they have osteoporosis until they suffer broken bones. These fractures, which usually occur in the spine, hip, or wrist, can be crippling or even fatal. Once you suffer a fracture, there is little that doctors can do to reverse the disease, and the risk of getting another injury jumps an incredible 20 times. The statistics are staggering. About 1.5 million Americans (most of them women) are victims of osteoporosis-related fractures each year. Few women realize that they are more likely to die from a hip fracture than from breast cancer.

The good news—and one of the main messages of this book—is that osteoporosis is very preventable in most women regardless of age. As researchers continue to unravel the secrets of estrogen, the main female sex hormone at the heart of so many changes in your reproductive life and health, they are rapidly expanding what is known about how and why bones weaken. New tests and medications such as Evista are also available that make it easier to tailor preventive measures and treatment options to your specific needs. If you are approaching menopause or especially if you have moved beyond it, it is important for you to learn as much as possible about osteoporosis and to assess your risk. In this chapter we will peer beneath the skin, deep into the little known but surprisingly active lives of bones. You will learn how bone cells, calcium, and hormones interact on an invisible level to help determine your bone health.

Q: What is osteoporosis?

A: The term *osteoporosis*, derived from the Greek for "porous bones," is used to describe an age-related, gradual weakening of the bones that causes them to become more fragile and vulnerable to potentially debilitating fractures. Doctors refer to this as a loss of bone density (also referred to as a loss of bone mass), because osteoporotic bones are literally less dense and strong than are healthy bones. This loss of bone density and decay in structural integrity make bones lighter and more porous. This means that they are less capable of bearing normal weight and break much more easily. In fact, a woman with osteoporosis may fracture a bone in a slight fall or even by stepping off a curb! Although 90% of people with osteoporosis are postmenopausal women over age 50, the process by which your bones begin to lose density usually begins in your twenties due to low calcium intake, too little exercise, and an unhealthy lifestyle. See Chapter 2 for information on preventing osteoporosis.

Q: Are there different kinds of osteoporosis?

A: Actually, there are several. Most women with the condition have type 1 osteoporosis, also called postmenopausal osteoporosis. It almost always strikes women and occurs primarily due to loss of estrogen during menopause. This is the kind of osteoporosis that you most often read about in newspapers and magazines or hear about in the news. Type 2 osteoporosis, also called senile osteoporosis, affects both men and women over age seventy. Women are twice as likely to have the disorder. Doctors also make a distinction between primary and secondary osteoporosis. The term *secondary* is used to describe osteoporosis that is caused by medications that you may be taking or by other medical conditions. Otherwise osteoporosis is referred to as *primary*.

Q: What are my bones made of?

A: When most of us think about bones we conjure up images of rattling, Halloween-type skeletons or the chalk-white, seemingly indestructible bones that dogs are always burying in cartoons. These images are misleading. Our bones are very much alive. They are living, breathing structures in a constant state of change. Understanding how and why bones change is an important first step in learning why osteoporosis occurs and how it can be prevented.

The basic ingredients that make up bones are minerals, proteins, and sugars, among other substances. There are two main types of bone: hard, compact bone and spongelike bone. It may help to picture the cross-section of a bone (a bone neatly cut in half, lengthwise) in order to better understand the way it is built. The outer layer or ring visible on the inside of the bone is made of hard and compact bone tissue—called *cortical bone*—and resembles a tube. This type of bone accounts for 85% of all bone in your body. Densely packed and capable of bearing great weight and stress, the hard, compact type of bone is well suited to support muscles and protect organs. It also houses the material within it.

Inside the tube of hard, compact bone lies the spongelike, porous bone that is filled with tiny hollow spaces. The spongelike type of bone, called *trabecular* bone, makes up the other 15% of bone. This type of bone is lighter and has an important shock-absorbing quality. Everyday walking and lifting, not to mention more strenuous activities, would be unbearably jarring without the presence of spongelike bone to cushion the impact. Not every bone in your body has the same amounts of hard, compact bone and spongelike bone; some have more of the first kind while others have more of the second. Although both types of bone may be affected by osteoporosis, the spongelike bone is usually affected first and to a greater extent. The vertebrae contain a large amount of spongelike bone and are the most common site of osteoporosis-related fracture. The hip contains both types of bone.

Q: Where does calcium enter the picture?

A: The building blocks of bone are made of calcium and other minerals such as phosphate. Bones also contain active cells called *osteoclasts* and *osteoblasts*. These cells are involved in the process by which bones grow stronger and denser or become weaker and brittle. The osteoclast group of cells resembles a biological wrecking crew. Their job is to remove the building blocks of calcium and other minerals from your bones—essentially removing bone, bit by tiny bit—and send them back into the bloodstream. The osteoblast cells are builders, not destroyers. While the osteoclasts are removing tiny bits of bone, the osteoblasts are busy filling in bone by removing calcium and other minerals from the bloodstream. Osteoblasts use these to create new building blocks in the spaces left behind by the wrecking ball of the osteoclasts. As your skin unceasingly sheds old cells for new, the more than 200 bones in your body are essentially being broken down and rebuilt constantly throughout life. Doctors refer to this dynamic process as bone remodeling.

Q: What does bone remodeling have to do with the strength or weakness of my bones?

A: You probably are not aware of it, but your bones are the scene of a never-ending contest between competing osteoclast and osteoblast cells. Whichever type of cell is able to do its job better—the osteoclasts that destroy bone or the osteoblasts that build bone—determines the health of your bones at any stage in your life by making them stronger or weaker. When the construction crew of osteoblasts is able to add more calcium to your bones than the osteoclasts can remove, as is the case during the first few decades of life, your bone density and strength increase. When bone loss exceeds the creation of new bone, your bone tissue loses density and becomes weaker and less healthy.

One of the major factors that affect bone remodeling is the amount of calcium available in your bloodstream.

Calcium is used by the body for purposes beyond that of bone building. If there is not enough calcium circulating in your blood to serve the heart, muscles, and nerves, the body will call upon the osteoclasts to remove the necessary calcium from your bones and divert it to these areas. At such times the osteoblasts may not be able to find enough calcium left in the blood to fill the gaps left by the missing building blocks. This negative calcium balance makes bone weaker.

Q: Is it true that my bones were stronger at age 30 than at age 18?

A: Surprisingly, the answer is yes. You may not have grown any taller after adolescence, but your bones continued to get stronger well into adulthood. If you plotted the strength of your bones on a chart, this is what you would see: The line representing your bone strength would move in an upward direction for the first 30 or so years of your life, then hold steady for a few years, and finally begin to turn downward. Most bone growth takes place during infancy and adolescence. During your teen years alone, 45% of total bone structure is created. After that, creation of bone continues to exceed bone loss—bone density increases—until you approach the third decade of life. Around that time, at about age 28, most women reach peak bone density for the spongelike type of bone, the type of bone most prone to fractures. Peak bone density is your maximum bone density—this is the state in which your bones are at their strongest. It varies from woman to woman. By age 35 a woman usually reaches peak bone density for the hard, compact type of bone.

Q: What is the significance of peak bone density?

A: In general, the higher your peak bone density, the lower your risk of developing osteoporosis later in life. The results of a number of twin studies as well as other evidence suggest that genetics play a major role in determining how much peak bone strength a woman has; in other words, mothers and daughters (and other close female relatives) tend to have a similar peak bone density. If your mother has strong, healthy bones, there is a good chance that you do too. The fact that blacks have an average bone density that is 10% to 15% greater than that of whites is also considered to be supporting evidence for a strong genetic role.

But heredity is not the only thing that determines your peak bone strength. Peak bone density can also be affected by a number of very controllable factors, including diet and exercise. Bone strength is often likened to a savings account: The more bone strength you have, the more you can afford to lose later in life when advancing age and other factors make withdrawals inevitable. Some doctors believe that young women can increase peak bone density by up to 20% (a sizable deposit) if efforts are made during the years crucial to bone building—from childhood to around age 30. A *New England Journal of Medicine* study reported that children receiving low dosages of calcium supplements attained higher peak bone density than those who did not receive supplements. This emphasizes the fact that it is almost never too early to begin taking steps to increase bone strength and reduce the risk of osteoporosis.

Q: Why does a woman's bone health get worse later in life?

A: The short answer is lack of estrogen, although a number of other factors come into play, including the normal tendency for aging bones to get weaker. After you have reached peak bone density, the creation and destruction of bone occur at equal rates for a while—the opposing forces of osteoclasts and osteoblasts are evenly matched—meaning that your bone density and strength remain about the same. But by your late thirties or early forties, the tireless osteoclasts have nudged ahead, and old bone is removed faster than new bone can be created. Your bones begin to get weaker.

At first, this loss of bone is not great. Then between ages 38 and 42 the production of estrogen by your ovaries declines and eventually stops altogether at the completion of menopause, which occurs roughly ten years later. Estrogen is a remarkable hormone. Among its other functions, it has a protective effect on your bone strength and health. When that protection begins to retreat, the loss of bone density speeds up. Some women suffer only a minor loss of strength and weight-bearing ability and maintain adequate bone health during and after menopause. But in women who develop osteoporosis, the loss of bone density is significant. Bones affected by the condition do not change much in size but become lighter, and the hollow spaces become larger, causing the bones to break more easily. A number of factors, discussed later in this chapter, influence whether or not you are at risk for developing osteoporosis. See Chapter 2 for more information on the different stages of menopause and associated rates of bone loss.

Q: What is estrogen?

A: Estrogen is the primary female sex hormone (men produce estrogen but in much lower amounts). Estradiol is the main estrogen and is produced in your ovaries; it operates from puberty to menopause. Measurements of estradiol are used to determine your estrogen level since estradiol is most often involved in conditions such as osteoporosis that are related to estrogen deficiency. Two other kinds of estrogen, called estriol and estrone, are also produced by your body, especially after menopause. Estrogen functions within a larger framework called your endocrine system—a complex biological network composed of organs and glands that secrete hormones to other areas of the body in order to regulate a variety of body functions. In women this network includes the ovaries, thyroid gland, pituitary gland, adrenal glands, pancreas, and hypothalamus. The various hormones help regulate reproduction and growth, digestion, bone building, calorie burning, body temperature, and metabolism. A hormone is like a chemical message carrier. Once produced by an organ or gland, it is sent through the bloodstream to a specific receptor on another organ or gland (into which it fits the way a key fits into a lock), where it either turns on or turns off—or speeds up or slows down—activity at the site. The way that estrogen stimulates, or fails to stimulate, activity in various parts of your body has significant effects on the maintenance of bone health and on other aspects of your health.

Q: Why is estrogen so critical to the health of my bones?

A: While there are many factors that may contribute to the development of osteoporosis, menopause is considered the most significant risk factor because this is the time in life when women lose the protective effects of estrogen. Estrogen and other hormones are largely responsible for regulating the bone-remodeling process. The link between osteoporosis and postmenopausal women was first discovered about 40 years ago when a doctor named Fuller Albright noticed that 40 of his 42 patients who had osteoporosis were postmenopausal women. Since then doctors have examined the role played by estrogen in maintaining the health and integrity of bones. They found that estrogen affects key aspects of the bone-remodeling process. It helps bone growth by stimulating the action of bone-building osteoblasts. It encourages calcium uptake by bone tissue and stimulates the activity of vitamin D. Vitamin D is manufactured by the body in response to direct sunlight and facilitates the body's absorption of dietary calcium (the calcium that you get from food or drink). Estrogen has effects on other hormones as well. It hampers the activity of parathyroid hormone, a hormone that tends to have a negative effect on bone strength; stimulates the production of calcitonin, a hormone produced in the thyroid gland that inhibits bone loss; and stimulates the liver to block the action of bone-weakening adrenal hormones. Estrogen may also stimulate the production of collagen, the framework upon which bone is deposited.

Q: Is it true that women often have lower levels of calcium and vitamin D in their bodies as they approach menopause?

A: This is true. You can think of calcium and vitamin D as the dynamic duo that fight bone loss. But this team is only effective if you have adequate amounts of calcium and vitamin D in your bloodstream. Unfortunately, as your body loses estrogen it becomes less efficient at absorbing dietary calcium and turning it into the building blocks of bone. This problem is made worse by the fact that most women do not get enough calcium in their diets to begin with. The body also tends to manufacture less vitamin D as estrogen levels go down, so less calcium is available for use by the body. Doctors sometimes prescribe calcium and vitamin D supplements for women during and after menopause to make sure that they have enough.

Q: What is the most serious consequence of osteoporosis?

A: The breaking of bones. Because osteoporosis is a silent disease and typically causes no symptoms, too often the first indication of it is a fracture. Although any bone may be affected, the vertebrae, hips, and wrists are particularly susceptible to osteoporosis and fracture because they contain a relatively high proportion of spongelike bone, which is lost earlier and more extensively than hard, compact bone. In extreme cases of bone deterioration a cough or suddenly coming to a stop while walking can cause a fracture.

Compression fractures (fractures of the bones of the spine) may lead to loss of height or to the stooped posture referred to as dowager's hump. Compression fractures often go unnoticed but can cause intense pain. About 40% of women will have at least one spinal fracture by the time they reach age 80.

Hip fractures are about half as common as spinal fractures, but they can be devastating. A woman's risk of experiencing a hip fracture is equal to her combined risk of getting breast, uterine, and ovarian cancer. About 20% of women who have hip fractures die within six months, and 10% to 20% die within a year. This occurs in part because a woman who has a severe fracture of the hip may be confined to bed for a long period of time, during which she is more vulnerable to blood clots, stroke, pneumonia, and other serious conditions.

If you already have had a fracture, your risk of another fracture is 25 times that of a woman who has the same degree of bone loss but who has not broken a bone.

By the time you fracture a bone, it is very difficult to make a major impact on the condition. Early diagnosis and preventive measures are the best ways to avoid fractures. See Chapter 3 for more information on fractures.

Q: What exactly is a risk factor?

A: A risk factor for osteoporosis is something that makes you more likely to get the condition. Generally, the more risk factors you have, the greater your chance of developing osteoporosis. Some of these risk factors are in your control while others are not. For example, you cannot change your age or race, but you *can* stop smoking. Your goal should be to cut your risk for osteoporosis as much as possible by targeting controllable risk factors that you can do something about. The major risk factors for osteoporosis are listed below. See Chapter 2 for more information on how to assess and reduce your risk of osteoporosis.

- ***Age.*** Your risk of developing osteoporosis increases with age. By age 65, the average woman has lost about 25% of her peak bone density.
- ***Race.*** Whites and Asians are more likely to get osteoporosis than are blacks. Genetic factors are thought to be the reason. Peak bone density on average is greater in blacks than in whites or Asians and this may explain why blacks suffer less from the condition. Some doctors think that whites and Asians process vitamin D—half of the dynamic duo—in a slightly different way that results in a lower peak bone density. A genetic advantage may have developed during evolution in races living in areas of strong year-round sunshine. As you saw earlier in this chapter, sunlight stimulates the pro-

Percentage of Osteoporosis in Different Age Groups of Women

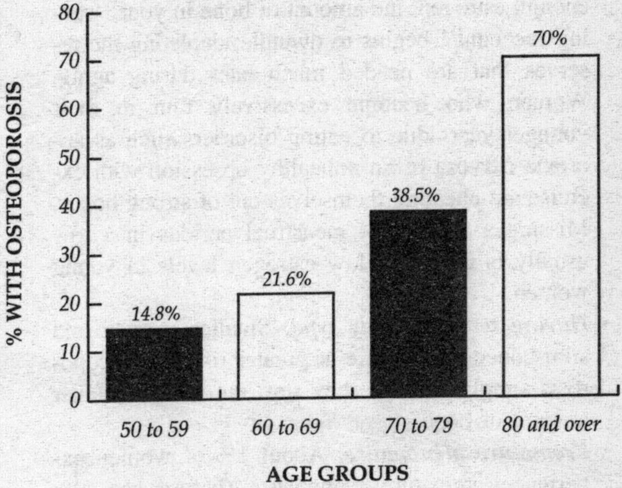

duction of vitamin D. People living in the northern hemisphere do not get as much sunlight on average.

- ***Family history.*** Osteoporosis runs in families. If you have close female relatives affected by osteoporosis you are at greater risk for the condition. Some women may carry a specific gene that makes them more likely to get osteoporosis, but this has not been proven. This gene may affect how the body uses vitamin D.
- ***Missed menstrual periods or being chronically underweight in your youth.*** Were you the sort of young woman who strove to emulate the gaunt look of a fashion model? If so, you have a greater chance of getting osteoporosis than a woman who maintained a healthy weight in her youth. A certain

amount of fat is necessary in order for your body to produce proper levels of estrogen. Without enough estrogen, the amount of bone in your "savings account" begins to dwindle, depleting the reserves that are needed much later during aging. Women who become excessively thin in their younger years due to eating disorders such as anorexia nervosa or an unhealthy obsession with exercise are cheating themselves out of strong bones. Missing a number of menstrual periods in a row usually is a sign of low estrogen levels in young women.

- ***Having a small body type.*** Smaller women and slim-boned women are at greater risk for osteoporosis simply because they start out with a smaller amount of bone.
- ***Premature menopause.*** About 1% of women experience premature menopause (before age 40). This can occur naturally or due to surgical procedures that involve removal of the ovaries. Not every type of surgery involving the reproductive organs causes surgical menopause. Simple hysterectomy—the removal of the uterus—does not cause early menopause. Procedures such as total hysterectomy (the removal of the ovaries as well as the uterus) do induce early menopause. Premature menopause can also occur due to damage to the ovaries by radiation or chemotherapy. If you smoke, you may experience premature menopause because smoking reduces estrogen levels. Early menopause is also associated with more frequent and severe hot flashes and with an increased risk of heart disease.
- ***Cigarette smoking or alcohol abuse.*** Alcohol contributes to the development of osteoporosis in sev-

eral ways. Protein deficiency associated with alcoholism can increase your risk. Heavy drinking, even when not linked to protein deficiency, may hamper the work of osteoblasts—the cells that help to build bone—and have a negative effect on the bone-remodeling process. Alcohol also interferes with the absorption of vitamin D. Smoking increases your risk for weak bones by reducing estrogen levels.

- ***Calcium deficiency.*** The modern diet is low in calcium. A latte in the morning is often all the calcium the busy American women gets. There is strong evidence that calcium deficiency is a contributing factor in the development of osteoporosis. As you saw earlier in this chapter, calcium is a key building block of bone. The osteoblast cells cannot keep your bones strong if you are not getting enough calcium. Many women with osteoporosis have trouble digesting dairy products, and this may explain why they had trouble getting enough dietary calcium. Studies of women living in foreign countries in which dietary calcium intake is low have an increased number of hip fractures and decreased bone density in the hard, compact bone. See Chapters 2 and 8 for more information on getting enough calcium in your diet.
- ***Vitamin D deficiency.*** New medical studies suggest that vitamin D deficiency may play a greater role in the development of osteoporosis than was previously thought. A 1998 study in the *New England Journal of Medicine* suggests that many Americans lack sufficient amounts of vitamin D in the blood needed to adequately protect against bone loss. In another study of 160 people between the ages of 49

and 83 who visited hospital clinics of the Boston University Medical Center, 40% were deficient in vitamin D. Vitamin D deficiency is attributed to insufficient dietary intake and inadequate exposure to sunlight. Increased use of sunblock during the summer has also contributed to decreased sun exposure.

- ***Inadequate exercise.*** Inactivity and lack of regular exercise, especially weight-bearing exercise, contribute to loss of bone. Astronauts actually have experienced some bone loss while in space. This occurred because they were in a zero-gravity environment in which they did not have to bear the weight of their own bodies. Despite the fact that American women are exercising more than ever, they still exercise less than men do regardless of age. Women also tend to exercise less as they grow older. See Chapter 8 for recommendations on exercise.
- ***Medications.*** Certain medications can lead to the development of secondary osteoporosis. These include thyroid hormone (used to treat hypothyroidism); corticosteroids (used to treat asthma and arthritis); phenytoin (Dilantin), an anticonvulsant; aluminum-containing antacids; and gonadotropin-releasing hormone, or GnRH (Lupron), used to treat infertility and endometriosis.
- ***Preexisting medical conditions.*** Hyperthyroidism, Cushing syndrome, diabetes, and kidney problems may also lead to secondary osteoporosis.
- ***Caffeine.*** Sorry, coffee lovers. High levels of caffeine (more than three cups of coffee a day) can reduce calcium levels and may promote bone loss if you do not get more calcium in order to compensate.

Risk Factors for Osteoporosis

- Being female
- Having a thin or small frame
- Advanced age
- A family history of osteoporosis
- Being postmenopausal or having had early or surgically induced menopause
- Amenorrhea (abnormal absence of menstrual periods)
- A diet low in calcium
- Use of certain medications
- An inactive lifestyle
- Cigarette smoking
- Excessive use of alcohol
- Being white or Asian, though blacks are at significant risk as well

2

Preventing Osteoporosis

Quick Fact: Studies show that many women get less than half the calcium required for maintaining healthy bones.

Jennifer, age 22, is a flight attendant. One day after aerobics class she noticed a pain in her foot. After three weeks her foot was still painful. A visit to the orthopedist revealed a stress fracture in her right foot. Jennifer was worried. She was certain she had osteoporosis. Her doctor reassured her that was not the case since stress fractures are not typical for osteoporosis. Jennifer did weight-bearing aerobics four days a week and drank three glasses of milk every day. However, she often dieted severely, and it was not unusual for her to go several months without a menstrual cycle. This meant that her estrogen levels were low—low enough to possibly weaken her bones. Jennifer's doctor referred her back to her gynecologist, who told her that being underweight and missing periods put her at risk for osteoporosis later in life. Jennifer went on a low-dose oral contraceptive to boost her estrogen levels, cut back on ex-

ercise to three days a week, and began to have normal menstrual cycles.

The fact that half of all postmenopausal women eventually develop osteoporosis is disappointing to doctors because they know that osteoporosis is easily preventable. It is almost never too early to craft a personal strategy of prevention and to educate the youngest women in your life about osteoporosis so that they can begin taking steps toward building healthier bones. But an individualized approach is essential when it comes to prevention. The best strategy to prevent bone thinning depends on your age, your medical history, your calcium intake, how much estrogen (if any) is being produced by your ovaries, and whether or not you have risk factors.

In your younger years, prevention largely consists of eating right and staying fit in order to make bones stronger. It is during these years that the bone-friendly, construction-worker cells called osteoblasts are busy creating new bone by extracting and laying down building blocks of calcium and other minerals that circulate in the blood. You can make their job a lot easier by getting enough calcium in your diet and by stopping bad health habits that contribute to bone loss. If you strengthen your bones early in life, they will return the favor in years to come by being strong and resilient when the wrecking crew team of cells called osteoclasts starts working overtime to destroy bone.

As you get older, the focus shifts to preserving the amount of bone that you have. If you are approaching menopause or have already completed it, you and your doctor will work together in assessing the health of your bones—painless bone density testing, for example, can be used to measure your bone density—and devising the best ways to maintain bone health. You can play your part by being an informed and active partner in your own health care and by choosing the best combination of preventive options that your doctor has to offer. In some cases this means only a program of diet and exercise—and possibly calcium or vitamin D supplements—and occasional monitoring by your doctor. But your strategy may also include powerful medications such as Evista (raloxifene) that are proven to put the brakes on bone loss.

Q: What advice do you have for a younger woman who wants to prevent osteoporosis?

A: If you are a younger woman, you are in a great position to increase the strength of your bones. The best time to build bone strength is between childhood and age 30. Your preventive strategy during this time should consist of getting adequate dietary calcium (calcium from food or drink), doing regular weight-bearing exercise, and eating a nutritious diet. Avoid carbonated drinks, which often contain caffeine and other substances that interfere with the absorption of calcium. Try to get 15 minutes or so of sunshine every day, which is necessary to stimulate your body's production of vitamin D. (Be aware that sun exposure can put you at risk for skin cancer, so be sure to wear sunscreen to protect yourself against the harmful effects of ultraviolet rays if you are planning on spending time in the sun.) You probably do not need vitamin D supplements at this age. In fact, too much vitamin D can actually cause bone loss. The 400 international units (IU) of vitamin D typically found in multivitamins is an adequate amount to prevent osteoporosis in this age group and will not cause bone loss. It is also important to make healthy lifestyle choices when it comes to smoking or your use of alcohol and caffeine.

An overall program of proper diet and exercise has

many other health benefits as well. It may reduce your risk of heart disease and cancer, melt away stress, and improve your mood. You should remember that even at this age it is not too early to talk to your doctor about osteoporosis. Your doctor can tell you if you have risk factors for the condition, help you design a diet and exercise regimen, and also offer practical advice for stopping smoking and eliminating other unhealthy habits. See Chapter 8 for in-depth information on the basics of eating right and staying fit. Here are a few things that you can do right now to start making your bones stronger and reduce your risk of osteoporosis:

- ***Get enough calcium.*** Calcium is a key building block used by osteoblasts to make bones stronger. If you do not get enough calcium (which is usually found in dairy products), your body will remove this building block from bone for use in other parts of the body, leaving you with less stored bone strength—the total amount of bone strength that you have before bones begin to lose density around age 35 or so. If you are lactose intolerant (have a problem digesting dairy products) it is important that you get calcium from nondairy sources or calcium supplements. Some good sources of calcium from various food groups include 1 cup of plain, low-fat yogurt (415 mg); 1 cup of skim milk (302 mg); 1 oz of cheddar cheese (204 mg); ½ cup of cooked broccoli (136 mg); and 3 oz of sardines with bones (370 mg). See Chapter 8 for more information on good sources of dietary calcium.
- ***Get off the couch and exercise!*** Exercise can increase bone density. Your exercise regimen should balance weight-bearing exercises with activities that

get your heart pumping. Though many women lift weights these days, weight-bearing exercises do not necessarily involve pumping iron in a sweaty gym. Walking, jogging, racquet sports, hiking, aerobic routines, jumping rope, bicycling, and stair climbing are weight-bearing activities as well. The trick is to experiment with different kinds of exercise until you find those that you enjoy and that you can do on a regular basis.

- ***Do not smoke.*** You may already know that smoking increases your risk of heart disease and cancer and is linked to numerous other health problems. Smoking also increases the likelihood that you will get osteoporosis later in life. Smoking interferes with the processing of vitamin D, which in turn means that you will absorb less calcium. Smoking also leads to early menopause and lowers circulatory estrogen levels, which also increases your risk. Talk to your doctor about strategies that you can use to kick the habit. There are also a number of helpful devices on the market for stopping smoking; ask your doctor about which products would be suitable for your needs.
- ***Do not drink.*** Stop drinking alcohol or limit yourself to two drinks a day—less if possible. Even a little alcohol can interfere with how your body absorbs and processes calcium and vitamin D. Drinking too much alcohol also goes hand in hand with other unhealthy habits; chances are that if you are drinking heavily you are probably not getting enough exercise or eating properly either.
- ***Avoid caffeine.*** Do you depend on a couple of cups of coffee every day to keep you going? If so, you may be increasing your risk for osteoporosis. Caf-

feine causes your body to lose calcium. Stop drinking coffee or tea altogether or try to drink less than three cups of coffee or tea a day. You may also want to try drinking a mixture of decaffeinated and regular coffee and then gradually reducing the amount of regular coffee that you add.

- ***Relax.*** While a certain amount of stress is unavoidable, too much stress can interfere with the absorption of calcium and speed up the release of adrenal hormones. These hormones make osteoclasts, the cells that destroy bone, work harder. If you feel overstressed, talk to your doctor about stress management techniques.

Q: I have recently been diagnosed with osteoporosis and I know that the condition runs in families. Is there anything that I can do for my ten-year-old daughter to keep her from getting it later in life?

A: Yes. In fact, there are many practical things that you can do. Educate your daughter and other young women in your life about the importance of bone health, which is something they may not be thinking about very much. You can encourage healthy habits in them even before they are old enough to really understand what osteoporosis is or why it is important to prevent. You can do this in a couple of ways. Make sure that your daughter is getting enough calcium in her diet and that her diet is well balanced and nutritious. Explain to her why it is important to eat right and be active and set an example yourself. Do not discourage her from the running and jumping that is typical of the play of young children. Encourage your daughter to play games or sports that require her to be physically active. Researchers have found that up to half of all children do not exercise on

Recommended Calcium: Are You Getting Enough?

Women under age 25	**mg/day**
Ages 1 to 10	800 to 1,200
Ages 11 to 24	1,200 to 1,500
Women over age 24	
Pregnant and lactating	1,200 to 1,500
Ages 25 to 49 (premenopausal)	1,000
Ages 50 to 64 (postmenopausal taking estrogen)	1,000
Ages 50 to 64 (postmenopausal not taking estrogen)	1,500
Over age 64	1,500

Source: Adapted from the National Institutes of Health Consensus Panel, Optimal Calcium Intake, 1994.

a regular basis. It may help to find an activity that you and your daughter can do together.

As she gets older, make sure that your daughter understands that there is such a thing as being too thin and exercising too much. Be on the lookout for any signs of an eating disorder—such as anorexia nervosa—or the use of fad diets. These can be particularly destructive because the loss of estrogen that occurs in a woman with an eating disorder can result in lower peak bone density, and peak bone density is an important indicator of who gets osteoporosis and who does not. If you spend a little time teaching your daughter healthy habits while she is young, chances are that she will carry those habits into adulthood and that they will become a regular part of her life. It is much harder to unlearn bad habits in adulthood than it is to learn the basics of proper diet and exercise early in life.

Q: Girls seem so thin these days. What is anorexia and how can I tell if my daughter has it or is just slim?

A: Good question. An anorexic is often very skilled at hiding her problem, so you will need to learn the warning signs to figure out if your child is among the 5% to 10% of young women between ages 12 and 18 who have full-blown anorexia or milder forms of the condition. In simple terms, anorexia is an obsession with thinness that goes beyond normal dieting. Anorexics have a distorted body image (they think that they look fat even when they are wire thin) and an abnormal need to control food. The typical anorexic is usually of high school age—a high achiever involved in sports such as gymnastics, swimming, cheerleading, or ballet. In addition to weight loss (an anorexic may lose 25% of her body weight in a few months), exercising too much or too often is typically one of the earliest signs. Anorexics often feel cold even when the temperature of a room is normal because their overly thin bodies cannot maintain heat. They complain of cold feet and their teeth are often sensitive to heat and cold. Most anorexics stop having menstrual periods. Physical weakness, energy loss, sleepiness, failure at school, and fainting spells may all be subtle indications of the disorder. Anorexia is a serious medical condition that requires a doctor's care.

Q: I am a woman in my early forties. I know that bones start losing density faster when menopause starts, but how will I know for sure when menopause has started?

A: The truth is that many women do not realize that menopause has started until it is already under way. Menopause is not a single event—you do not simply stop having menstrual periods overnight—but a gradual process that can last up to ten years. Menopause occurs on average around age 51 (most women experience it sometime between ages 46 and 56). The process of menopause—and the speeding up of bone loss—begins years earlier. The first stage is called *perimenopause* (which means "around the time of menopause"). Perimenopause refers to the several years leading up to menopause itself, which occurs when menstrual periods have stopped for a period of 12 months in a row. It can be a little confusing because the word *menopause* is often used (as it is used in this book) to include the perimenopausal stage as well as the point at which menstrual periods stop completely. When menopause is complete, your ovaries have stopped producing estrogen and you are officially a postmenopausal woman.

The experience of menopause is different for each woman. You may experience menopausal symptoms right away, as you enter the perimenopausal stage, or you may be included in the 25% of women who sail through menopause from beginning to end without suffering any troublesome symptoms. The women who have the least trouble with menopause—some women even welcome the change—are those who respond to it in an informed and active way. Some symptoms that you may experience at the perimenopausal stage are irregular periods, missed periods, mild hot flashes (sensations of heat in the neck, chest, or face) the day before a period, and an increase in premenstrual syndrome (PMS) symptoms. As you approach menopause itself, your menstrual periods will get further apart until they eventually stop altogether. Due to the loss of estrogen during menopause, you may experience a variety of symptoms. The number and severity of these symptoms—and whether you experience them at all—vary from woman to woman. These symptoms include hot flashes (about 75% of American women experience them fairly early in the process and they may continue for several years after menopause is complete), night sweats, difficulty sleeping, shrinkage and dryness of the vagina (which can result in uncomfortable sex), skin problems (dry skin, acne, or sensitivity), urinary tract infections, and moodiness or a feeling of depression. See Chapters 6 and 7 for more information on how to treat menopausal symptoms.

Q: How much bone density can I lose during menopause?
A: You begin to lose bone density in your late thirties and early forties, but this loss of bone speeds up during and immediately after menopause. During menopause you may lose 3% to 5% of your bone density per year. You lose the most bone during the first five or so years after menopause. Then, about six to ten years into the postmenopausal stage, the rate of bone loss goes down to somewhere around 1% to 3% per year, although some women continue to lose bone faster than that. You may lose a total of 25% of your spongelike bone and 10% of your hard, compact bone just as a result of estrogen loss. Unfortunately, that is not the whole story. During

the same time that you are rapidly losing bone density because of a lack of estrogen, your hard, compact bones are also slowly getting weaker due to the natural march of time. What does all this add up to? In your lifetime, you may lose up to 35% of both the spongelike bone and the hard, compact bone that you had at your peak. In many women this bone loss leads to osteoporosis. That is why it is so important to take steps to make bones stronger while you are young and to prevent bone loss if necessary when you get older.

Q: When is the best time to talk to a doctor about my risk for osteoporosis?

A: If you are approaching menopausal age or have experienced any symptoms of menopause, talk to your doctor about osteoporosis if you have not done so already—especially if you have any of the risk factors described in Chapter 1. After all, no one cares more about your health than you do, and many doctors are uninformed or unfamiliar with preventive care. Informed patients usually make the best decisions about their health, and your doctor will appreciate the fact that you are taking an active role in your own care. This sort of open communication often results in a more productive partnership between you and your doctor. Before talking to your doctor, you may wish to take a brief osteoporosis risk quiz (see below). This will help you assess your risk for the condition and make you better prepared to answer questions during your exam.

Q: What can I expect during my visit to the doctor?

A: Your doctor will review your medical history (this will probably include a series of questions designed to help evaluate your risk), give you a physical exam, and prob-

Osteoporosis Risk Quiz: How do you score yourself?

(Your risk increases with each yes answer.)

1. Does osteoporosis seem to run in your family or are there older women in your family who seem to fall a lot?
2. Are you white or Asian?
3. Did you miss periods when you were younger or have an eating disorder?
4. Do you have a small frame or have you always been very thin?
5. Did you experience menopause early, whether naturally or due to surgery?
6. Do you smoke or drink a lot of alcohol or caffeinated drinks?
7. Do you have trouble digesting dairy products?
8. Have you spent most of your life not getting much exercise?
9. Have you taken medication for hypothyroidism or arthritis for long periods of time?
10. Have you ever been diagnosed with hyperthyroidism, Cushing's syndrome, diabetes, or kidney problems?

ably recommend a bone density test. Osteoporosis is impossible to detect early on by a physical exam. Only when irreversible damage has occurred is it visible to the examining doctor. The bone density test usually is performed in a hospital or other facility. A bone density test measures your bone mineral density (BMD) so that it can be compared to that of an average woman your age and size who does not have osteoporosis or to the estimated peak bone density of a healthy woman.

Not all doctors agree about when bone density testing is called for. Some doctors recommend a bone density test for any woman around the age of menopause while others may only suggest it if you have risk factors or are postmenopausal. Bone density testing is also used to monitor how well you are responding to measures taken to prevent bone loss, such as medication treatment. You should ask your doctor's opinion about bone density testing during your visit. The fact remains that a bone density test is the most reliable way to evaluate the health of your bones at any point in time. Many health care companies now pay for part or all of the cost of preventive bone density tests if you have one or more risk factors for osteoporosis. Check with your insurance company to be sure. Your doctor may also recommend certain blood and urine tests to further evaluate your risk of getting osteoporosis and to rule out other conditions that may be causing bone loss. Urine tests are used to determine how well your body is processing calcium and if you are losing bone density rapidly. Blood tests measure calcium levels and estrogen loss, provide clues to bone formation, and indicate whether your body is processing nutrients effectively.

Q: What sorts of tests will a doctor use to assess my bone health and osteoporosis risk?

A: Tests that measure bone density are the primary methods used by doctors to evaluate the integrity of your bones. These tests are used for several purposes: to detect osteoporosis before the occurrence of a fracture, to predict your risk of fracture in the future, and to determine your bone loss rate or monitor the effects of treatment (on an annual basis). Most of these tests, which are all safe and painless, measure BMD in your hip, spine, or wrist—common fracture sites. The cost of getting a bone density test varies but the average is about $150, with the exception of the Sahara Clinical Bone Sonometer test (see below). Dual energy X-ray absorptiometry (DEXA) takes only a few minutes and is usually the method of choice when a BMD measurement is required. DEXA exposes you to a low level of radiation—about the same amount of radiation exposure you get on a coast-to-coast airline flight. Urine tests that measure the byproducts of bone breakdown may also be used as an indicator of bone deterioration.

Computed tomography (CT) scans are sometimes used to measure BMD but they use more radiation than other techniques and are more expensive. Other tests include dual photon absorptiometry (DPA)—a procedure that assesses the total calcium and mineral content of your hip and spine but that uses more radiation—and single photon absorptiometry (SPA), which is usually used to measure the amount of the hard, compact bone. There are also blood tests that aim to measure bone formation, and new blood tests are being developed that assess the extent of bone destruction by attempting to measure osteoclast levels.

The Sahara Clinical Bone Sonometer, a new BMD measuring device that does not use radiation, was approved for use by the Food and Drug Administration (FDA) in early 1998. This test uses ultrasound—high-frequency sound waves—to assess the integrity of your bones by measuring the density in your heel. The cost of the bone sonometer test (about $40) is less than half that of a DEXA procedure and appears to be just as effective.

A BMD measurement is not always an accurate indicator of your risk and is not done in every case.

Q: What is a bone density test actually like?

A: Bone density tests are noninvasive. Your body will not be penetrated (or even poked and prodded) during the test. You do not have to stop eating or watch what you eat before the test and in most cases you do not have to remove your clothing. Most bone density tests, which do not take long and in some cases are over in a few minutes, measure BMD by passing a stream of radiation through one or more bones. More or less of the radiation will pass through the bone depending on how dense the bone is. If the bone is dense, less radiation passes through it. If the bone has low BMD, more radiation is absorbed by the bone and less of it passes through. Unlike other bone density tests, the Sahara Clinical Bone Sonometer does not use radiation at all; it uses sound waves to measure your BMD.

During a bone density test, you will be in a sitting or lying position depending on which part of your body is being evaluated. If your heel or wrist is being measured, you will be seated in a chair and your heel or wrist will be allowed to rest on a specially designed support where it will be tested. If your spine or hip is being measured, you will lie on top of a scanner table. A device beneath the table will send radiation upward, where it will pass through tissue and bone; another device located above the table will measure how much radiation has passed through. A CT scan is a little different than the other bone density tests. During a CT scan, you will lie on your back on the top of a table. This table is then moved into a large hollow space in the shape of a tube, where the test itself is done. It sounds more frightening than it actually is, but if you have a fear of tight, closed-in spaces you should discuss this with your doctor before having a CT scan done.

Q: Is one sort of bone density test better than another?

A: DEXA is considered the gold standard of bone density tests by most doctors and will probably be recommended if it is available in your area (it may not be). Although it is more expensive than SPA or DPA, DEXA uses less radiation than most bone density tests, can measure bone density at the three most common sites of fracture (hip, spine, and wrist) in minutes, and gives the most accurate measurements of spongelike and hard, compact bone. DEXA measures bone density directly at the sites where fractures typically occur. Many doctors use DEXA to measure the bone density in the hip and spine because fractures in these areas are common and often debilitating. Some doctors believe that a bone density measurement of the heel or forearm bone gives an accurate measurement of the bone density throughout the body. This single-site method of determining bone density is usually done using SPA or the Sahara Clinical Bone Sonometer. Whether this single-site method of testing is as good as directly measuring the density of the hip, spine, or wrist is a matter of controversy among doctors.

Q: What is the meaning of the phrase *fracture threshold* and why is it important?

A: *Fracture threshold* is a phrase used by doctors to describe a BMD measurement that is dangerously low. If your BMD falls just below the fracture threshold, your risk of fracturing a bone is about two times that of a woman who has healthy bones. If your bone density is lower than it should be but has not yet reached the fracture threshold, the term *osteopenia* is used to describe your condition. If bone loss is allowed to continue, you will develop clinical osteoporosis, which occurs when your BMD falls below the fracture threshold. Frequently, however, the term *osteoporosis* is used to describe a woman with low bone density even if her BMD is above the critical fracture threshold. The *exact* definition of osteoporosis is not as important as identifying women with low bone density early and taking steps to prevent further loss of bone.

Q: What is the next step after testing?

A: The results of bone density and other tests help your doctor to evaluate the state of your bones. Based on these findings and your medical history, you and your doctor will design a preventive strategy tailored to your specific needs. Keep in mind that a single bone density test does not necessarily tell the whole story. Just because your bone density is healthy at the time of testing does not mean that it will remain that way. Your doctor may want to test you again in the future. By comparing later tests with earlier tests, your doctor can see how quickly you are losing bone. For the bone-healthy woman, however, annual scans may be excessive and testing may not need to be repeated at all if new therapy is started after a recheck scan.

If your bone density is low (but not too low) and you are menopausal, medication such as Evista may be recommended after menopause is complete to prevent further weakening of your bones. If your bone density is low enough, estrogen therapy may be recommended premenopausally if irregular menstrual periods have begun. No matter what testing reveals, the preventive strategy that you and your doctor create will include healthy eating habits and weight-bearing exercise. Your doctor will also consider whether or not you need calcium or vitamin D supplements, which often can be taken along with other medication.

Q: I have been tested and found to have low bone density, but I have not yet reached menopause. What are my treatment options?

A: Your doctor cannot prescribe Evista until you have reached menopause. However, in addition to making sure that you maintain a healthy lifestyle and exercise regularly, you may be a candidate for treatment with estrogen replacement therapy (ERT) or hormone replacement therapy (HRT). ERT and HRT use a form of estrogen made in a laboratory to replace estrogen lost during menopause. ERT or HRT given during the first few years of menopause can delay or prevent the development of osteoporosis—in fact, there is an 85% chance that with ERT or HRT you will prevent bone loss. There are risks associated with estrogen therapy, including the possibility of cancer of the breast or uterus. The risk of uterine cancer associated with ERT is reduced sharply by adding the hormone progesterone to estrogen therapy—it is referred to then as HRT. Doctors cannot agree if ERT and HRT encourage the development of breast cancer. In some studies estrogen therapy appears to increase the risk of breast cancer while in others it does not. ERT and HRT have many other beneficial effects in addition to slowing bone loss. They reduce the number and severity of many of the symptoms of menopause and may reduce the risk of heart attack by up to 50%. See Chapter 7 for more information on estrogen therapy.

Q: I am already postmenopausal. Is there anything that I can do to prevent osteoporosis at this point in my life?

A: Absolutely, assuming that you do not already have the condition. But because half of all postmenopausal women eventually develop osteoporosis, it is important to talk to your doctor now in order to develop a strategy of prevention or to start treatment. (See your doctor right away if you experience sharp, steady pains in your upper and middle back—these may be symptoms of fragile bones that are just beginning to fracture.) Being a postmenopausal woman does not automatically mean that you have dangerously weak bones. You may be surprised to find that you have the bone density of a woman in her twenties, in which case your preventive program may simply consist of a diet and exercise regimen and maintaining proper levels of calcium and vitamin D. If medication is necessary, you have several choices in addition to ERT or HRT. These medications are described briefly below.

- ***Evista***. This hormonal medication was approved by the FDA in late 1997. A selective estrogen receptor modulator (SERM), Evista is designed to act like estrogen in some parts of the body while blocking its effects in others. It does not slow bone loss quite as well as estrogen does but it has not been associated with breast or uterine cancer. Evista may even reduce the risk of heart disease and breast cancer, although it has not yet been approved by the FDA for those purposes. See Chapters 4, 5, and 9 for more information on Evista and other SERMs.
- ***Alendronate (Fosamax)***. A nonhormonal medication, alendronate is the strongest bone-building product on the market. It works by slowing the ac-

tivity of the osteoclasts—the biological wrecking crew team of cells that destroys bone. Alendronate is often used in women who cannot or choose not to take ERT or HRT, although doctors are studying the effectiveness of taking alendronate and estrogen therapy together. See Chapter 7 for more information on alendronate.

- ***Calcitonin (Calcimar or Miacalcin).*** A hormonal medication taken to prevent osteoporosis, calcitonin is available as an injection (Calcimar), but most women choose the nasal spray form (Miacalcin). It is for use in women five years after menopause and is usually recommended for women who cannot or choose not to take one of the medications mentioned above. Calcitonin is not as strong as estrogen therapy or alendronate, but it has the fewest side effects of any of the medications and reduces pain in women with osteoporotic spine fractures. See Chapter 7 for more information on calcitonin.

3

Living with Osteoporosis

Quick Fact: Fifty percent of women over age 50 will suffer a fracture due to osteoporosis.

Greta, age 73, works as a secretary at a travel agency. She lives on her own and is fiercely proud of her independence. One day she was standing on the bus when it came to a very sudden stop. Although she did not fall, an hour later she noticed an intense pain in her middle back that wrapped around her ribs. For days she could not sleep. Her daughter finally convinced her to go to the emergency room. X rays showed two compression fractures in her upper spine. The doctors at the hospital prescribed Greta a codeine-containing medication that relieved the pain, but Greta became so confused by the effects of the medication that she could not care for herself. I helped Greta put her suddenly out-of-control life in order. I stopped her narcotics and began nonsteroidal medication. I also prescribed calcitonin, a medication that increases bone density in the spine and also helps to ease pain. Greta was sent to a physical therapist, who placed a transcutaneous electric nerve stimulation (TENS) unit on her back that almost immediately began to relieve her pain. The physical therapist also taught her to do exercises to strengthen her back. After three weeks Greta was back on the job and working hard to strengthen her bones and prevent further fractures.

Whether you are picking up your grandchild for the first time or lifting a bag of groceries, stepping into the bathtub or even opening a window, osteoporosis can affect the cherished moments in your life as well as your everyday activities. The millions of women in America with very low bone density are at much higher risk of experiencing a bone-breaking injury than are women with healthy bones. Many of these fractures result from falls—something that older women are prone to—while others can happen simply by stepping off a curb. But having osteoporosis is no reason to retreat fearfully from the world around you. By learning as much as you can about the condition, you can work with your doctor to fashion a long-term plan to minimize the effect of osteoporosis on your life.

There is no cure for osteoporosis, no magic pill to restore your bones to the condition that they were in before you were diagnosed with very low bone density. But your doctor has a growing arsenal of powerful medications such as Evista that are effective at preventing further bone loss and making your bones stronger. Once you have been diagnosed with low bone density, it is crucial to preserve every ounce of bone that you have. Bone density testing allows your doctor to peek inside your bones from time to time to see how well your treatment plan—which will also include dietary therapy and an exercise regimen—is working and to make changes if necessary. Your doctor will explain how painkilling medications, acupuncture, transcutaneous electric nerve stimulation (TENS), and heat or massage therapy can be used to ease some of the aches and pains associated with osteoporosis.

But medication is not the whole story. Understanding how fractures occur and doing everything you can to prevent them is a major part of staying healthy when you have osteoporosis. It does not take much force to fracture a weakened bone. The sorts of accidents that might leave other women with only a bruise can cause serious injuries in women with low bone density. There are a number of reasons why women tend to fall more as they get older. The side effects of your blood pressure medication, a problem with your eyesight that you have not sought care for, even your favorite shoes—these and a number of other factors can make you a little less steady on your feet.

Q: What is the most serious kind of fracture?

A: You are standing on tiptoes in the kitchen, straining to reach up into a high cabinet where you keep the flour. You feel around for it—you know it is in there somewhere. Suddenly your foot slips and you fall backward onto the hard surface of the newly washed floor, landing squarely on your hip. Too often situations like this introduce women with osteoporosis to the most serious type of fracture—that of the hip. About 300,000 of these fractures occur each year, and they are ultimately responsible for the deaths of 50,000 women annually. When not fatal they rob thousands of other women of their ability to live on their own or to lead independent and active lives. A hip fracture is not the most common type of break; however, most women are surprised to learn that if they combined their risk of getting breast, uterine, and ovarian cancer, it would equal their risk of having a hip fracture.

Q: Who gets hip fractures and why are they so serious?

A: Hip fractures almost always occur in women over age 50—about 50% of them happen to women over age 80—whose bones have been weakened by osteoporosis. The typical victim is white; blacks get hip fractures less often, probably because they tend to have a higher peak bone density. Twenty percent of women who suffer hip fractures due to osteoporosis die within one year. For women in their seventies and eighties who suffer hip fractures, the statistics are even more alarming—up to half die within a year after the fracture.

At first you may not see how a fracture can actually be life threatening. After all, you may have had a broken bone yourself when you were younger and been back on your feet (and no worse for wear) before everyone had a chance to sign your cast. But the bones that typically break due to osteoporosis are not the same as those you may injure in your younger years, and the consequences are more serious. A hip fracture itself is not immediately fatal. The reason that hip fractures can be deadly is that a woman who has a severe fracture of the hip often receives long-term medical care or hospitalization that makes her vulnerable to other conditions such as blood clots, stroke, or pneumonia, among others. These happen as complications of surgery or as a consequence of being confined to bed for a long period of time.

Q: How do hip fractures usually happen?

A: Like many bone-breaking injuries due to osteoporosis (vertebral fractures being a major exception), hip fractures are usually the result of falls—perhaps in the shower or kitchen or on an icy sidewalk. Most women (90%) break their hips by falling onto a hard surface from standing height or even lower. The woman who suffers this type of fracture typically lands directly on her hip without anything to break her fall. Usually not even fat or muscle cushions the blow because as women age they tend to have less of both. Studies show that about 50% of these falls are the result of slipping and 20% to 30% occur because a woman loses her balance; as you will see later in this chapter, many falls can actually be prevented with a little forethought. Once a hip actually fractures, the treatment—which can be very costly—is usually hospitalization, surgery (which may involve the placement of an artificial joint), and months of sometimes painful therapy. The cost of all this amounts to tens of thousands of dollars.

Q: How exactly does a hip fracture rob women of their independence?

A: As the front line of medical science advances against some of the most common afflictions associated with aging—such as high blood pressure, heart disease, and dementia—more and more women are able to lead fruitful and active lives well into their sixties and seventies and beyond. Many women today take pride in living on their own during their senior years without being heavily dependent on others. You probably have a relative or friend who comes to mind or you may be one of these women yourself. Unfortunately, a hip fracture often changes this situation virtually overnight.

Fifty percent of women who suffer hip fractures are never able to walk as well as they used to and many cannot walk without some sort of aid. This loss of ability radically alters how these women live and what they are capable of doing. Thirty percent of women with hip fractures become very dependent on others in order to function on a day-to-day basis. Women who once treasured their independence must turn to family and friends to aid them or else live in nursing homes or other facilities. According to one statistic, of women with hip fractures who used to live independently before the injury, almost 25% are still in long-term care institutions a year after the break.

Q: If a hip fracture is the most serious type of fracture, what is the most common type?

A: Vertebral fractures, also called compression fractures, are at the top of the list. More than 700,000 of these fractures occur every year, and by age 80 almost 50% of women have had one. Unlike hip and wrist fractures, vertebral fractures do not usually occur during a fall. This makes early diagnosis and treatment especially important because preventing falls may not protect you from a vertebral fracture.

Q: How do vertebral fractures happen?

A: It usually does not take much force for a very weak vertebra to fracture. As bones become thinner and weaker due to osteoporosis, the weight of the body while standing or walking may be enough to cause a fracture, as may bending or lifting. You can fracture a vertebra by simply lifting a bag of groceries, opening a window, or stepping off a curb. A vertebral fracture may go unnoticed but it often causes severe back pain—the kind of pain that makes it difficult to stand, walk, or lift. Even sneezing or coughing can cause pain in some cases, and a vertebral fracture can also disrupt sleep. If you have a vertebral fracture you may need to rely on the help of others until you can resume normal activities, which usually occurs a couple of weeks after the fracture. You may be left with a chronic dull ache in the back or neck. In the case of a severely curved spine, breathing may be uncomfortable.

Q: Do vertebral fractures make women shorter?

A: They can. In fact, osteoporosis is the most common cause of getting shorter with age, though after your mid-forties you begin to lose a small fraction of your height every year. Because one fractured vertebra can cause a ¼ inch loss of height, a couple of these fractures can make you shorter by several inches. The stooped posture of dowager's hump is often the result. Dowager's hump results when the spine is bent forward due to fractured vertebrae.

Q: Where else could I have a fracture?

A: Wrist fractures are pretty common, and it is easy to see why. Bending the wrist is a common reflex that we use to catch ourselves as we start to fall or to actually break a fall and prevent a more serious injury. More than 200,000 wrist fractures occur every year and they are usually the result of trying to break a fall. A fracture of the wrist can often be treated on an outpatient basis, and it is not as serious as a hip or vertebral fracture. Physical therapy is usually required and your doctor will discuss exercises that you can do at home. Another 300,000 or so fractures occur each year in other bones in the body, such as the shoulder or pelvis. Fractures in these bones usually result from falls as well.

Q: Do older women really fall more often than younger women?

A: This is no myth—older women actually do fall more than do their younger counterparts, and the consequences on health are usually more serious. While you may not hear much about it, falling is a major problem for older women and it has taken on almost epidemic proportions. As incredible as it sounds, in an average year almost one in three people over age 65 fall. Of people over age 80, almost one in two will fall at least once. In seniors, accidental deaths are ranked sixth overall and most of these involve falls. For a woman with osteoporosis, falling can be debilitating or fatal.

Q: Are older women just clumsier?

A: No—clumsiness has little to do with it. There are a variety of reasons why women fall more as they get older. Fortunately many of these falls can be prevented. Older women tend to fall due to muscle weakness and poor coordination, medication side effects, environmental hazards, existing medical conditions, or the effects of alcoholic beverages. Almost anything that causes dizziness, drowsiness, or disorientation can make a fall more likely. Here are some other reasons why older women are prone to falls:

- ***Vision problems***. Vision worsens with age. Nearsightedness, farsightedness, cataracts, or glaucoma can change the way you see and make you more likely to fall. You may need more time to adjust to sudden changes in lighting. Your peripheral vision and depth perception may also be affected as you age. You should have regular eye exams to detect any problems.
- ***Slowed reflexes***. Your reflexes tend to slow as you grow older. Exercise can help. Take your response time into consideration during your daily activities

and allow yourself to take more time with certain tasks if you find that it is necessary.

- ***Loss of hearing***. Being able to hear well is important to staying oriented and alerting you to danger. If you think that you may be losing your hearing, talk to your doctor about getting a hearing test; you may need a hearing aid.
- ***Loss of feeling in the feet.*** Loss of sensation in the feet can occur due to diabetes, vitamin D deficiency, or alcohol use.
- ***Arthritis of the knees, ankles, and hips.*** Stiffness or abnormal gait prevents people with arthritis from regaining their balance.

Q: Do most fractures occur in the winter?

A: Yes, most fractures occur during the winter months. Doctors have even pinpointed the time of day when most fractures occur—in the afternoon. But *where* most fractures occur may surprise you. Most bone-breaking injuries due to osteoporosis do not occur on icy sidewalks or streets. Most happen indoors. Some doctors think that due to lack of direct sunlight, many women suffer from vitamin D deficiency in winter (which would hinder their body's ability to absorb dietary calcium) or that some sort of neuromuscular deficit makes some women less steady on their feet.

Q: How can the pills that I am taking make me more likely to fall?

A: Your doctor prescribes medication with good reason—to improve or preserve your health and quality of life. *You should never stop taking medication or take more or less of it without talking to your doctor first.* But as you probably know, every medication has its side effects. Ironically, certain medications taken to improve your health can cause side effects—such as drowsiness, dizziness, disorientation, and slowed reflexes—that can actually make you more likely to fall. These include sedatives, antidepressants, muscle relaxants, tranquilizers, heart or blood pressure medication, diuretics, and sleeping pills. If you take more than one of these medications (or a large dosage of one), you may be more affected by the sort of side effects that lead to unsteadiness. Make sure that any doctor who prescribes medication for you knows that you have osteoporosis. You and your doctor can discuss medication options and ways to minimize your risk of falling.

Medications with Side Effects That Make Falls More Likely

Sedatives/ Tranquilizers	Antidepressants	Antihypertensives
flurazepam (Dalmane)	amitriptyline (Elavil)	methyldopa (Aldomet)
diazepam (Valium)	doxepin (Sinequan)	clonidine (Catapres)
	imipramine (Tofranil)	
	haloperidol (Haldol)	

Q: Can exercise help to prevent falls?

A: Yes. This is yet another wonderful benefit of exercise. No matter what your age, exercise can build muscles and improve balance, reflexes, and coordination, making falls less likely or less serious. But if you have osteoporosis, do not strap on those running sneakers or dust off those barbells in your attic just yet. As you will see later in this chapter, it is important to talk to your doctor first and to make sure that you do only those exercises that are safe for you.

Q: Where do I start when it comes to preventing falls?

A: Your home is a great place to begin. It may seem strange to think that you can injure yourself seriously in the home that you feel so comfortable in and in which you have lived for years. It is a lot easier to see the dangers posed by stepping off a curb in order to cross an icy street. But the fact is that most falls occur indoors. By evaluating your home for risks and taking a few simple steps, you can greatly reduce your risk of falling. As you will see, most of the precautions that you should take to prevent falls are based on common sense. Take a good look around your house and think about your daily routine. Which rooms do you tend to use and what do you do in them? What are the routes that you usually take? By reviewing the safety information below and thinking about your own personal habits, you will soon be able to think of plenty of other ways to make your home a lot safer.

The first step is to identify the danger areas. As you might expect, the bathroom is considered the most dangerous room in the house when it comes to falls—not just because it is easy to slip in the bathroom but because it has a large area of hard surfaces that are unforgiving to the bones. The tub or shower can be a dangerous place at any age, but women with osteoporosis are especially vulnerable to the consequences of falling there. Who has not slipped in the bathroom at least once or come awfully close to it, regaining balance at the last moment?

Q: How do I make the bathroom a safer place?

A: The best way to make your tub or shower safe is to install safety bars. A combination of bars can be placed on the walls enclosing your tub or shower to provide you with support—something to hold on to—while taking a shower or bath and stepping into or out of the tub. You may hesitate at first at the idea of installing bars in your bathroom. This is understandable, no one wants her home to resemble the cold and clinical atmosphere of a hospital. Fortunately this fear is unfounded. These days safety bars can be custom-fitted and color coordinated to match your bathroom's interior. At $15 to $30 a bar, they are well worth the cost. They can be bought at your local hardware store or from a company that sells medical equipment. They can even be ordered by mail, though it is always a good idea to see what you are buying firsthand before actually purchasing it. After you have bought the bars, the next step is to install them properly. Remember that these bars can do their jobs—supporting the weight of your body—only if they are securely attached to the wall. Call a plumber or carpenter if you have any doubts about installing the bars safely and securely.

Q: Any other tips for the bathroom?

A: In addition to bars, some women benefit from the use of a bench or chair in the tub or shower. If you have trouble standing in the shower or standing up or sitting down in the tub, a bath chair may be right for you. You should not use any old chair that you happen to have lying around the house—use only a chair that is specially designed for this purpose. These chairs are about twice the cost of a bar and usually can be bought at a medical equipment company. There are also certain bath benches available that are designed to extend out over the rim of the tub. They may look a little strange at first but can really be a help if you have a limited ability to move. Using a bench such as this, you can sit down on the part of the bench that is outside the tub and then slide over the bench to the part of it that is inside the tub itself. These benches cost around $100.

The final two safety tips for the bathroom involve mats and bath oils. Make sure that you have good non-skid mats or strips on the floor of the tub or shower to improve traction. This is important because the floor of the tub or shower can become very slippery. If your mats are old and have lost their grip, be sure to buy new ones—it is worth the investment. Bath oils can make the surface of the tub or shower even more slippery, so it is best not to use them. Try applying body oils instead, after leaving the tub.

Q: What else can I do to make my house safer?

A: In general, keep things in your home in easy-to-reach places so that you do not have to use stepstools or ladders to get them. The more trouble you have to go to in order to reach an object in your home, the greater your risk of slipping and falling in the process. Keep your high-traffic areas free of clutter or other obstacles that may cause you to trip. When you are in the kitchen, wipe up spills immediately and be especially careful when washing or waxing floors. It is probably a good idea to forego waxing altogether as an unnecessary risk. Here are some other tips for staying safe at home:

- ***Keep rugs firmly in place***. Just about everyone has slipped on or tripped over a throw rug. These rugs can either slip out from under your feet or a loose or floppy edge can make you trip. You can eliminate this risk by removing all throw rugs from your home. Otherwise, make sure that they are securely taped or tacked in place. Smooth out rugs if necessary to get rid of dangerous air bubbles that could cause you to stumble.

- ***Brighter is better.*** Are you in the habit of wandering into the bathroom or kitchen in the middle of the night without bothering to turn on the lights? If so, you are not alone. You probably figure that you know the way well enough and you do not wish to wait for your eyes to adjust to the bright light. However, when you have osteoporosis, it is not worth the risk of tripping over unseen obstacles or taking a wrong turn. Also, keep in mind that night vision decreases with age. One solution is to install a few nightlights in hallways and stairways—making sure that commonly taken routes are well lit. This way you will be able to see just where you are going (and what is in your path) when making a late-night trip to the bathroom or to the kitchen for a midnight snack. It is also a good idea to keep a flashlight next to your bed so that you always have a source of light should you need it; make sure that the batteries are fresh. The lighting in other rooms of your house is no less important. The basic rule: You should always be able to turn on the lights of a room by hitting a switch just inside the doorway. The idea is to avoid stumbling through the darkness in order to turn on a lamp or overhead light whose switch is on the other side of the room. Voice- or sound-activated lamps are also available. Using 100-watt bulbs will make it easier to see any clutter or potential obstacles in your path.

- ***Wear the right shoes***. Do not wear slippers with thick soles (especially those that your foot slips out of easily) or high-heeled shoes. Both can make you a little unsteady, especially if something upsets your balance. The shoes that you wear should have nonskid soles. Soles made of fabric may cause you to slip. Socks and stockings are notoriously slippery. It is an altogether different story now than during childhood, when you probably enjoyed getting a running start and sliding across the kitchen floor in your socks.
- ***Keep stairs safe***. Be sure that all stairwells are well lit and have rails on both sides. You may wish to put fluorescent tape on the edges of the top and bottom stairs to make them easier to see.
- ***Stay in touch***. If you live alone, you are probably proud of your ability to get by with as little assistance as possible from others. The best way to protect that independence is to make sure that you stay in touch with a friend or relative who does not live with you. There are several ways that you can do this. Some women choose to carry a cellular phone around with them in their homes. These phones are so small that they can fit into a pocket, and they serve a dual purpose: They allow you to answer the phone wherever you happen to be in your home and also make it possible to contact someone for help if you need it. It is important to stay in daily contact with your friends or loved ones. Make it a part of your daily routine—a social break. It is a good way to maintain relationships and to make sure that someone will know that something may be wrong if you do not call. There are also monitoring companies that will respond to your call 24 hours a day;

Quick Tips for Preventing Falls Indoors

Bathroom. Place safety bars and nonskid mats in the tub or shower. Do not use bath oils.

Kitchen. Place nonskid mats in front of the sink. Wipe up spills immediately. Be especially careful when washing or waxing the floor.

Lighting. Install nightlights in halls and stairways, especially along the routes you take during late-night trips to the kitchen or bathroom.

Stairs. Be certain that rails and rugs are secure. Place fluorescent tape on the edges of the top and bottom stairs to make them more visible.

General tips. Remove rugs, or tape or tack them down securely. Remove clutter from high-traffic areas. Wear low-heeled shoes and avoid slippers that are platform-like or that have fabric soles.

you probably will need to wear a small electronic device that you can use to call for help should you need it.

Q: How can I prevent falls when I am outdoors?
A: Here are some precautions for staying on your feet.

- ***Use canes or walkers.*** Do not give in to vanity! Canes and walkers can do a great deal no matter what the weather conditions to make you more stable when you are on the go.
- ***Do not forget your feet.*** Whether indoors or outdoors, making smart footwear choices is important.

Always wear low-heeled shoes with good traction. In winter, wear comfortable boots with rubber soles that grip.

- ***Take the road less traveled.*** If the sidewalk looks slippery, walk on the bare grass instead.
- ***Bring your own salt.*** This next tip may sound a little strange, but it is effective and just goes to show how helpful a little forethought can be. When you go out in winter, take along a little bag or container of cat litter (cat lovers may be a little more at ease in handling this) or rock salt. You can carry it right in your pocket or in the glove compartment of your car. Sprinkle it on a surface that looks icy. The highway department uses salt on roads; there is no reason that you cannot apply the same principle on a smaller scale.
- ***Keep the area around your house safe.*** Survey the area around your house in order to make sure that it is risk free. Check your driveway and walkways for cracks or bumps and have them repaired promptly. Make sure that any stairs leading up to your porch (or other entrances) have rails on both sides and that these rails are secure. The pathway or route leading up to the front door should be well lit at night.

Q: I caught the exercise bug a little late in life, but I have really come to enjoy my workout. Now that I have osteoporosis, is exercising off limits?

A: You will be glad to hear that you can almost always continue to exercise, which is a good thing, because exercise is too important to eliminate from your routine unless circumstances absolutely forbid it. Besides its effects on bone, exercise can strengthen your muscles, improve your coordination and balance, and make you more flexible. These benefits make you less likely to fall or more able to prevent a fall from becoming a serious injury. Still, great care must be taken when exercising with very low bone density. Only your doctor can adequately say what level of exercise is right for you. Your doctor knows your medical history and what medications you may be taking, and these are important factors in shaping a workout program.

You cannot necessarily follow the same exercise regimen that you and your doctor devised when trying to prevent osteoporosis—doing this may actually cause an injury. It is especially important to consult your doctor if you have suffered any sort of fracture, particularly a hip fracture or a recent vertebral fracture. But even after you have experienced an injury, your doctor will encourage you to begin exercising as soon as possible at a level that is safe for you. Exercising with osteoporosis usually involves a walking program, strength-training exercises (for the hips, back, thighs, and arms), and exercises to improve balance and coordination.

4

Evista and the New Selective Estrogen Receptor Modulators (SERMs)

Quick Fact: Sales of Evista are expected to reach $200 million in its first year on the market and may climb to $1 billion in the next five years. The amount of money spent on osteoporosis medications in the United States may rise from $2.8 billion in 1998 to as much as $4 billion in the year 2000.

Marion, age 52, had not been to a doctor in three years before coming to see me. She had just completed menopause in the past year and had decided to take care of her health after years of what she referred to as "low maintenance." Menopause had gone smoothly; Marion had had few or no symptoms such as hot flashes, sleeplessness, or vaginal dryness. But she smoked half a pack of cigarettes a day and weighed 40 pounds over her ideal body weight. Both her parents had died of heart disease in their late sixties. Her mother suffered a heart attack the day after repair of a hip fracture.

Marion was obviously at increased risk of osteoporosis and heart disease. She thought her weight protected her against osteoporosis—"Isn't osteoporosis only a problem for thin women like my mother?" she asked—which is a common misconception. We discussed lowering her health risks, beginning with stopping smoking. Because she was at risk for both heart disease and osteoporosis, and because she did not want to be bothered with the possibility of menses or bleeding from hormone replacement therapy (HRT) after such an uneventful menopause, Marion decided to go on Evista once daily along with supplemental calcium. By her next visit she had quit smoking and had lost 10 pounds by starting a program of regular exercise.

The story behind the exciting new osteoporosis medication Evista (raloxifene) and the new breed of selective estrogen receptor modulators (SERMs) reads something like a chapter in a detective novel. Doctors played the role of sleuths, continuing to unlock the secrets of the hormone estrogen and putting existing hormonal medications under the magnifying glass in a search for clues—clues that led to a new kind of hormonal therapy: custom-made, estrogen-like medications that have all the benefits of estrogen without many of the potentially harmful effects.

For years doctors have known that estrogen affects various parts of the body in different ways. In bone and cardiovascular tissue, for example, estrogen has a healthy influence, helping to build bone and prevent heart disease. But in the breast and uterus, the effects of estrogen in postmenopausal women can increase the risk of cancer. The risk of breast cancer has only been demonstrated in women who have used estrogen for more than 10 years. The risk of uterine cancer exists primarily in those women who have not taken the uterine protective hormone progesterone. Despite the fact that estrogen replacement therapy (ERT) offers a variety of benefits for women after menopause—from easing hot flashes and vaginal dryness to preventing osteoporosis and heart disease—only 20% of postmenopausal women actually take estrogen, mainly due to fears that its effects on the breast and uterus will lead to cancer. While hormone replacement therapy (HRT) sharply reduces the risk of uterine cancer by including a cycle of progesterone along with replacement estrogen, many women simply are not willing to take the chance.

As is often the case in the world of science, the possibilities of Evista as an osteoporosis medication became the focus of intense scientific scrutiny almost by accident. The events that led to the appearance of Evista in American pharmacies in early 1998 were sparked years earlier while doctors were studying another SERM called tamoxifen (Nolvadex). You may have already heard of tamoxifen. It is the most widely used medication for the treatment of breast cancer. In late 1998 tamoxifen was approved by the Food and Drug Administration (FDA) for reducing the risk of breast cancer in women who are likely to develop the disease due to family history or other reasons—the first medication ever to make such an exciting claim.

In the early 1990s tamoxifen played a key role in the recent development of Evista and other SERMs when doctors discovered that tamoxifen acts like an estrogen in some parts of the body while blocking its effects in others. Because tamoxifen works as an anticancer medication by blocking estrogen's effect in the breast—where estrogen can have an unhealthy effect—researchers assumed that it would block estrogen's effect in the bones as well, causing them to lose density and become brittle. To their surprise they found that tamoxifen promoted bone growth and also had a healthy effect on cardiovascular tissue because it acts like an estrogen in those parts of the body. Unfortunately, tamoxifen also acted like an estrogen in the uterus, where the hormone can have an unhealthy effect and increase the risk of uterine cancer.

But the discovery that tamoxifen could act like an estrogen in certain parts of the body and block its effects in others created a renewed interest in other SERMs, the chemical cousins of tamoxifen. The hunt was on for a SERM that mimicked estrogen in just the right way—acting like estrogen in the bones and in cardiovascular tissue where it has a healthy effect but doing just the opposite in areas such as the breast or uterus. Theoretically, this SERM would offer protection against osteoporosis and heart disease without putting women at risk for cancer.

Evista, known at that time by its generic name raloxifene, was one of the first candidates. A SERM, it had been studied by its current manufacturer Eli Lilly as a possible anticancer medication in the 1980s but had never been investigated as a form of hormonal therapy for osteoporosis and heart disease. After studying the clues revealed by tamoxifen, doctors were able to shine a light on the full potential of Evista. Several years later, after being tested on thousands of postmenopausal women all over the world and earning approval by the Food and Drug Administration (FDA), Evista became the first of the new SERMs to become available to the public. As of early 1999, at least seven other SERMs were being studied by various pharmaceutical companies for the prevention and treatment of conditions ranging from osteoporosis and heart disease to cancer.

Q: What is Evista?

A: Evista is a new prescription medication used to prevent and treat osteoporosis in women who have completed menopause. Evista may not be used by women who are still having menstrual periods because it has not been studied thoroughly enough in this group. Evista has been proven to increase bone density—though not quite as much as ERT, HRT, or the nonhormonal medication alendronate (Fosamax)—and appears to have very few serious side effects in the short term when used properly. Studies have shown that it may also prevent breast cancer and heart disease, although the FDA has not yet approved Evista for these purposes. Evista and other SERMs are sometimes referred to as designer estrogens or second-generation estrogens because they mimic some of estrogen's effects but not others. See Chapter 9 for more information on whether Evista can help prevent heart disease and breast cancer.

Q: How do Evista and other SERMs work?

A: Evista and other SERMs represent a breakthrough in the effort of medical science to go one better than nature by designing chemical copycats of estrogen that imitate only the hormone's health-promoting qualities. As you saw in Chapter 1, estrogen acts like a chemical message carrier, speeding along the bloodstream and making stops at various destinations. These destinations are receptors located on the cell membranes of organs and glands throughout your body. By fitting into a receptor the way a key fits into a lock, estrogen delivers its messages by activating genes inside cells. The content of these messages has a tremendous impact on your health and well-being because the messages can affect reproduction and growth, digestion, bone building, calorie burning, the regulation of body temperature, and metabolism. Evista, tamoxifen, and other SERMs are also able to bind with the estrogen receptors. But SERMs are designed to act in specific ways at each of the receptor sites. In some tissues, a SERM may turn on the same genes as estrogen. In others, it may not. Sometimes doctors can measure the effect that a medication has without being able to explain exactly how it works. This is true to some extent with SERMs. Researchers are still studying how SERMs produce their effects.

Q: How do you take Evista?

A: You must take a tablet of Evista every day in order to help prevent osteoporosis. Once you stop taking it, you lose its protective effects over time. This is generally the case with osteoporosis medications. Because most women live one-third of their lives after menopause is complete, you may have to take Evista for years—perhaps decades—to stave off the loss of bone that leads to osteoporosis. Because Evista has only been studied in postmenopausal women for about two and a half years, the long-term effects of using the medication are not well understood. Women taking Evista should still take calcium and vitamin D supplements when needed and follow a diet and exercise regimen prescribed by their doctors.

Q: How effective is Evista?

A: Evista has been shown to increase bone density by about 2% to 4% in postmenopausal women. By way of comparison with other FDA-approved medications for osteoporosis, ERT and HRT generally increase bone density by 4% to 5% and alendronate has been shown to increase density by as much as 8%. During the approval process, the FDA reviewed studies involving almost 13,000 women from 28 countries to establish the safety and efficacy of Evista in the prevention and treatment of postmenopausal osteoporosis. The testing is far from over. Evista will likely continue to be studied for years to come in order to verify that it is safe and to understand how well the medication works in postmenopausal women and in younger women.

Q: Does Evista help to prevent fractures?

A: Because Evista is a new medication, there have been no studies that show whether or not it will actually reduce your risk of fracturing a bone due to low bone density. Most doctors think that it will, because increasing bone density usually helps to prevent fractures. Studies are now under way to find out in a more direct way if women using Evista are less likely to break a bone; these studies involve almost 8,000 women worldwide.

Q: Is Evista totally free of side effects?

A: Every medication has side effects—prescription and over-the-counter medications alike. In the case of Evista, side effects were reported as mild by most women in the studies. The most common complaint was an increase in the number of hot flashes. Evista did not increase the severity of hot flashes, just the frequency. Most women who experienced an increase in hot flashes while taking Evista continued taking the medication; less than 2% of women in the studies stopped taking Evista because of this side effect. The increase in hot flashes usually went away after about six months of using Evista. There have also been reports of stomach upset and a slight increase in leg cramps. These cramps were gen-

Who Should Not Take Evista?

- Women who have not completed menopause.
- Women who are on ERT or HRT (it is okay to start on Evista after stopping ERT or HRT).
- Women who have or have had blood clots in the legs, lungs, or eyes.
- Women who are or may be pregnant (Evista may harm the fetus).

erally reported as being mild in nature. Evista did not cause irregular spotting or bleeding or breast pain or tenderness, which are some of the common complaints of women taking estrogen.

Q: What about more serious side effects?

A: A rare but serious side effect of taking Evista is a blood clot in the legs, lungs, or eyes. Blood clots can result in significant health problems—potentially even death. This side effect is more likely to happen in women who are already at risk for clots in the first place. If you have blood clots, a history of blood clots or heart attack, or are overweight or confined to bed, you should discuss the risk of blood clots with your doctor before using Evista. Because Evista has only been tested for a few years, whether or not Evista has any serious long-term side effects is largely unknown.

Q: I remember hearing something in the media about Evista and ovarian cancer. Is that something I should be worried about?

A: No, not according to the FDA. Women taking Evista do not appear to be at higher risk for ovarian cancer or other problems of the ovaries. In studies, postmenopausal women taking Evista were no more likely to develop ovarian cancer than were women taking placebos. The media reports that you are probably thinking of were based on findings in rats and mice. The FDA determined that the findings in these rodents do not translate into a risk for people.

How Evista Affects Different Parts of Your Body

	Bone	**Breast**	**Heart**	**Uterus**
Evista	Acts like estrogen; has a healthy effect.	Blocks the effects of estrogen; appears to have a protective effect.	Acts like estrogen; appears to have a healthy effect.	Does not act like estrogen; appears to have no effect.

Q: Is Evista just another kind of estrogen therapy?

A: Definitely not. Although Evista and other SERMs are hormonal medications, they are different from ERT and HRT both in terms of chemistry and in their effects on your health. Evista and SERMs are chemical copycats, designed to masquerade as estrogen when it is useful and to put a roadblock in front of the natural estrogen produced by your body in order to prevent disease. Estrogen replacement, on the other hand, is a way of restoring the estrogen that your body has lost due to menopause. It does not make decisions about when to act like estrogen and when not to.

ERT and HRT are as close as medical science has come to finding a single medication that meets the various challenges to health and well-being posed by the loss of estrogen due to menopause. ERT and HRT can be used to ease the symptoms of menopause and to prevent or treat serious conditions that women are often more susceptible to as they grow older. Estrogen therapy can ease hot flashes, night sweats, and vaginal dryness. It maintains strong bones and reduces the risk of heart disease more effectively than any single medication approved for postmenopausal women. Recent research also indicates that ERT and HRT may reduce the incidence of Alzheimer's disease, and they certainly improve the mood and memory changes seen at menopause. Evista does nothing to ease menopausal symptoms (in fact, it slightly increases the number of hot flashes), nor does it have any effects—healthy or unhealthy—on brain function. Its effects on bone and cardiovascular tissue are also less strong than those of ERT or HRT.

But fewer than 20% of the almost 40 million postmenopausal women in the United States stay on estrogen therapy for a long period of time. ERT is associated with an increased risk of uterine cancer, and both ERT and HRT may increase the risk of breast cancer. (Despite numerous studies on estrogen therapy and breast cancer risk, doctors do not agree on whether or not ERT or HRT poses any threat to breast health.) Estrogen therapy can also cause breast tenderness, weight gain, and vaginal bleeding. Like Evista, the effects of estrogen therapy disappear once you stop using it, in which case rapid bone loss resumes and the cardiovascular protection begins to fade. Although estrogen therapy has been studied for 50 years, doctors are still learning new lessons about its safety and effectiveness.

Q: How does a medication get approved by the FDA?

A: When a medication such as Evista is approved for use by the FDA, that means it has met this federal government agency's standards for safety and effectiveness for certain and particular therapeutic applications. The overall process leading up to approval involves several stages of testing. This process typically takes years to complete and has a price tag of millions of dollars, which is paid by the pharmaceutical company that is trying to bring the medication into the marketplace. In early stages, testing is confined to lab animals such as mice, rats, and monkeys, in whom the effects of the medication are studied. If a medication clears this hurdle, it is later given to a small number of people. These volunteers are carefully monitored in order to determine if further testing on a larger group of people is justified. In the final stages, large-scale tests, called double-blind trials, are carried out in which neither doctors nor study participants know who is getting the medication as opposed to a placebo; this is done to make the test as objective and unbiased as possible. Once the FDA is satisfied that a medication works and is safe, it gives the pharmaceutical company that is sponsoring the medication the right to market it under a brand name. The pharmaceutical company then has the exclusive right to sell the medication until the patent runs out in 20 years.

Q: Is FDA approval a guarantee of safety?

A: Not exactly. FDA approval is a very important indication of whether or not a medication works and is safe for specific problems. But FDA approval does not mean that a medication is right for everyone to use or that a medication can be used safely for a long period of time. Even if a medication that you are thinking of taking is FDA approved, you should still find out as much about the medication as possible and weigh the risks and unknown factors in conjunction with your doctor. In many cases medications are approved by the FDA without knowledge of what the long-term side effects may be. Even if a medication has been approved by the FDA, it can still be recalled and pulled from pharmacies by the agency if it becomes clear that it poses a serious threat to public health.

5

Using Evista to Help Prevent or Treat Osteoporosis

> **Quick Fact:** One Evista (raloxifene) tablet should be taken every day in order to help prevent or treat osteoporosis.

Diana, age 50, is a busy executive who has always dreaded the idea of menopause. She had been treated by several doctors for the past four years for irregular uterine bleeding, but it seemed every treatment regimen she tried made her breasts unbearably tender or caused heavy bleeding. Yet Diana had always taken an active role in her own health—watching her cholesterol, exercising regularly, and keeping stress to a manageable level. She wanted to be equally proactive about her health risks after menopause but also wanted to avoid the daily discomfort that she associated with estrogen replacement therapy (ERT). Somehow she felt that her current healthy lifestyle was not going to be enough to keep her healthy as she got older. When Diana came to see me, her exam was normal, but to better address her current menopausal health I decided a bone density test was in order. The test surprisingly showed that Diana had lost bone density despite a healthy lifestyle. When she discovered that Evista had no significant impact on breast tissue and would not cause the breast tenderness or heavy bleeding that she had experienced previously on estrogen therapy, she agreed to start on Evista. A year later she felt great, and a follow-up bone density test showed a bone mineral density (BMD) increase of 3%. Menopause was not the dreadful event she had feared!

Before deciding whether or not to make Evista a major part of your bone-building strategy, discuss with your doctor the potential benefits and risks of using this new medication. You can play an active part in the decision-making process by getting as much information as possible about Evista and other medications used to fight bone loss. Ask as many questions as you need to of your doctor until you have a good understanding of what Evista may or may not do for you. Make sure that your doctor knows any and all of your concerns. Picking an osteoporosis medication is a personal decision that only you can make. Your doctor is there to help you make the choice that is right for you. Here are a few factors to consider and discuss with your doctor.

- ***Safety***. If you have breast or uterine cancer in your family, or if you are especially concerned about this type of cancer, it will be of particular importance to you that in two and a half years of testing, Evista has been shown to build bone apparently without increasing the risk of these cancers. Talk to your doctor about the most recent scientific thinking on the safety of Evista, and read Chapter 10 to find out how you can stay up to date on the latest Evista news.

- ***Effectiveness***. Evista is a powerful bone-building medication, but it does not increase bone density quite as well as estrogen replacement therapy (ERT), hormone replacement therapy (HRT), or the nonhormonal medication alendronate (Fosamax). If you have very low bone density, you and your doctor may need to take steps to strengthen your bones as much and as quickly as possible in order to prevent a potentially dangerous fracture.
- ***Side effects.*** Evista's side effects are generally mild, and most women in the studies did not stop using the medication due to these sorts of problems. While Evista may cause some estrogen-like side effects such as headache, bloating, and an increased risk of blood clots, it does not cause breast pain or tenderness the way that ERT or HRT can in some women. It also does not cause the spotting or menstrual-type bleeding that is sometimes a complaint of women receiving estrogen therapy.
- ***Evista's other possible healthy effects***. Evista appears to help keep the heart healthy, a major concern of women in their postmenopausal years because heart disease kills more women over age 50 than any other cause. Evista may also help to prevent breast cancer. The Food and Drug Administration (FDA) has not yet approved Evista for either of these purposes. Talk to your doctor about how much weight to give these possibilities in making your decision.

You may have been surprised to discover that some of the symptoms that gave you trouble during menopause did not end with last your last menstrual period. This is perfectly normal. After menopause, your body only has about 20% of the estrogen it had when you were younger, and this loss of estrogen may cause hot flashes, night sweats, vaginal dryness, and other symptoms. They affect most women to one degree or another and can last well into the postmenopausal years. Unlike ERT or HRT, Evista does not help to ease these sorts of problems and may even cause you to have hot flashes or more of them, at least for the first several months of use. If you choose to take Evista, you may need to find ways to ease these problems. You can combat them with the aid of prescription and over-the-counter (OTC) medications or with the alternative therapies used by many postmenopausal women. See Chapter 6 for more information on how to treat your menopausal symptoms while using Evista.

Q: How well will Evista work for me?

A: Because Evista is a new medication that only became available to the public in early 1998, most of what we know about it is drawn from medical studies involving women from the United States and other countries around the world over a period of several years. These are the same studies that the FDA examined during the approval process. While there is no way to guarantee exactly how well Evista will work for any particular woman, we can take a closer look at one of the major studies in order to see how other postmenopausal women fared on Evista. In this study, more than 500 North American women took 60 mg of Evista daily for two years. The average woman was age 54 and had completed menopause five years before starting on the medication. More than 90% of the women were white. (As far as doctors know, neither age nor race affects how

Evista works.) Some of the women were given Evista itself while others were given a placebo (sugar pill); all of the women in the study took calcium supplements as well. These women were examined after one year and again after two years to see if their bones had gotten stronger or weaker. This was a double-blind study, which means that neither the doctors who actually gave the women their pills nor the women themselves knew who was getting Evista and who was getting placebos. This helps to make sure that the testing is done in an unbiased and objective way.

Q: How did these women do?

A: In order to check the strength of these women's bones, doctors used a bone-density testing device called dual energy X-ray absorptiometry (DEXA) to measure how much bone had been gained or lost during the study. DEXA, which is discussed in Chapter 2, is the same kind of device that your doctor may use to check your own bone density. Doctors measured the bones of the hip and spine in these women. As you saw in Chapter 3, these are the bones that are most likely to break due to osteoporosis. The results of these fractures can be painful and debilitating—in some cases a fracture of the hip can be deadly. After two years, here is what the doctors found:

- ***In women who took Evista:*** Bone density in the hip went up by 2%. An increase such as this makes the bones of the hip stronger and healthier and less likely to break under the stress of a fall. When doctors measured another fracture-prone area of the hip called Ward's Triangle, they found that Evista had increased the bone density there by 3.1% to 4%. Bone density in the spine also grew by 2%, making the vertebrae stronger and less likely to collapse.

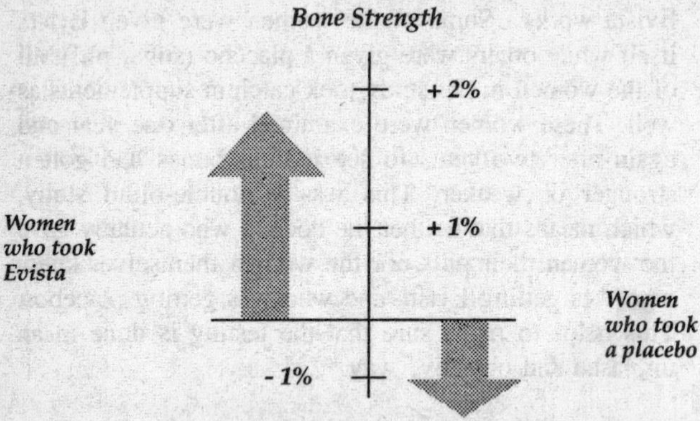

How Evista Strengthened Bone in a Test of More Than 500 Women

- ***In women who took placebos instead of Evista:*** Although these women took calcium during the study, they actually lost bone—about 1%. Without Evista, their bones continued to lose density during the study and got weaker.

So after two years, the women who took Evista had bone densities about 3% greater than those of the women who did not take Evista. Even after just one year, women taking Evista had stronger bones. Doctors cannot say for sure if these increases in bone density will help to prevent a woman from breaking a bone—more tests are being done to confirm that—but most doctors are confident that they will.

Q: How should I take Evista?

A: Evista comes in white tablets of 60 mg each. You should take one of these tablets each day. It makes no difference whether you take Evista on an empty stomach or right after you have eaten, and it also makes no difference what time of day or night you take the medication. Here is a tip: Although it is not required, it is often a good idea to take Evista at the same time each day. This will make taking your dose of Evista a part of your daily routine and will make it easier for you to remember. If you accidentally skip a day, there is no reason to be alarmed. Simply start taking the medication again on the following day according to your regular schedule. You should not take a double dose of Evista in order to make up for the one that you missed. For example, I had a patient who always took her Evista tablet first thing in the morning. That was the easiest way for her to remember to take it, before the hustle and bustle of her day really began. One morning she called to tell me in a worried tone that she had forgotten to take her medication the day before. I told her that it was not something to worry about and to go back to her regular schedule. But I also stressed the importance of taking Evista every day. If you do not take it regularly it will not be as effective at preventing or treating osteoporosis. Once you stop taking Evista, you lose its protective effects.

Q: Is it really as simple as just taking a pill once a day?

A: It is not quite that simple. You must remember that Evista or any osteoporosis medication is just a part of the long-term plan designed by you and your doctor to keep your bones as healthy as possible. While Evista is working to strengthen your bones, you can and should do plenty of other things. You should continue to take calcium or vitamin D supplements if prescribed by your doctor and eat a healthy diet. Exercise is another important part of your plan. If you have low bone density, you should only do the exercises recommended by your doctor. These exercises may vary depending on how strong your bones are at the time and if you are at high risk for a fracture. You should also avoid counterproductive, unhealthy behavioral habits that can contribute to bone loss, such as smoking or drinking too much alcohol or caffeine. Evista takes several months to one year before making any meaningful changes to your bone density. It is especially important during this time to understand what kinds of fractures you are most at risk for—the most common are those of the hip, spine, or wrist—and to take commonsense steps to avoid them. See Chapter 3 for more information on fractures and what you can do to prevent them.

Q: How do I know if Evista is safe?

A: Ultimately this is a personal decision that you must make in consultation with your doctor. The FDA has determined that Evista is safe when used properly. During the approval process, the FDA reviewed studies involving thousands of women worldwide. But even the FDA cannot guarantee that Evista is safe when used for long periods of time because the drug has only been studied for a few years. Because Evista is a hormonal medication that mimics some of the effects of estrogen, doctors were concerned that it may also increase the risk of cancer of the breast or uterus. As you saw in Chapter 4, estrogen therapy in postmenopausal women stimulates tissue in the uterus (when used without progesterone) and perhaps in the breast as well. This stimulation may encourage the growth of cancerous cells in some women.

Doctors agree that Evista did not appear to stimulate the breast or uterus in women who took it for about two and a half years. Whether or not Evista will increase the risk of breast or uterine cancer over a period of many years is largely unknown. As of early 1999, the test results were encouraging. Doctors will continue to test Evista and to monitor women who started on Evista years ago in order to confirm what they know about the safety of the medication. See Chapter 4 for more information on the FDA approval process and the safety of Evista.

Q: Who should not take Evista?

A: Evista is not recommended for every woman. It should only be used by women who have completed menopause and who are not on ERT or HRT. If you are still going through menopause, even if you have low bone density you cannot take Evista to make your bones stronger. You will need to consider using another medication instead. Here are some other cautions that you should know about.

- ***Blood clots***. You should not use Evista if you have blood clots or have had them in the past. These include clots in the legs, lungs, or eyes. Taking Evista may increase the risk of these clots, which can cause serious medical problems and even death. If there is anyone in your family with a history of blood clots, discuss this fact with your doctor before starting on Evista.
- ***Congestive heart failure (CHF) or cancer***. Women with either of these conditions are already more at risk for a blood clot. If you have CHF or cancer, you and your doctor will have to carefully weigh the potential benefits of Evista against the risks.
- ***Danger during pregnancy***. Evista should not be used in pregnant women because it may harm the fetus.

- ***A severe liver condition***. Evista has not been well tested in people with severe liver problems. In studies, women with cirrhosis who took Evista had 2.5 times more of the medication circulating in their bloodstream than did other women. If you have cirrhosis or another condition that affects your liver, you should talk to your doctor about whether or not it is safe for you to use Evista.
- ***Allergy***. You should not take Evista if you are allergic to it or to any of its other ingredients. While raloxifene is the active ingredient in Evista (the active ingredient is the main ingredient responsible for a medication's effects), Evista also contains a number of other ingredients called inactive ingredients. You should not take Evista if you are allergic to any of these. Be sure to tell your doctor about any allergies that you have.
- ***Smoking.*** Although women who smoke need the protective effects of Evista badly, smoking also increases the risk of blood clots and stroke. Quit smoking to protect your bones and preserve good health!

Q: Can Evista interact with other medications that I may be taking?

A: That is a good question, and the answer is yes. Like most medications, Evista has the potential to interact with other medications in ways that are unhealthy or even dangerous. It is very important that your doctor know about all the medications you are taking—especially prescription medications but OTC ones as well. When taken together, two or more medications sometimes have unwanted effects. Sometimes an interaction may make one or more of the medications that you are taking less effective; you may have to space these med-

Other Ingredients in Evista

- Anhydrous lactose
- Carnauba wax
- Crospovidone
- FD&C Blue No. 2 aluminum lake
- Hydroxypropyl methylcellulose
- Lactose monohydrate
- Magnesium stearate
- Modified pharmaceutical glaze
- Polyethylene glycol
- Polysorbate 80
- Povidone
- Propylene glycol
- Titanium dioxide

ications apart, adjust dosages, or change medications. In other cases certain combinations can cause dangerous reactions.

You should also talk to your doctor before taking any of the many alternative remedies available at your local pharmacy or health-food store. Although these products are sold over the counter and are often derived from plants, some of these products have powerful effects that mimic those of hormones or prescription medications. Only your doctor or pharmacist can tell you for certain what medications do not mix.

Q: What medications interact with Evista?

A: First of all, it is important to remember that doctors have not studied how Evista interacts with every medication on the market today. As more and more women begin to use Evista, more interactions may become known. From the medical studies that have been done so far, here is what we know now about how Evista and other medications interact.

- ***ERT or HRT***. You should not take Evista while you are on ERT or HRT. Doctors have not studied how these two hormonal bone builders interact in women.
- ***Ampicillin***. You should not combine Evista and ampicillin, an antibiotic sold under various brand names (D-Amp, Omnipen, or Polycillin, for example), because the interaction makes both medications less effective—less of each is absorbed by the body.
- ***Cholestyramine***. If you are on Evista and are also taking cholestyramine (Prevalite, Questran, or Questran Light), a medication used to lower cholesterol levels, you should take these medications at least one hour apart. The reason for this is that cholestyramine may reduce the amount of Evista absorbed by your body by 60%.
- ***Warfarin***. Evista may reduce the time it takes your blood to clot if combined with the blood-thinning medication warfarin (Coumadin, Panwarfin, or Sofarin). If you take Evista and warfarin, your doctor may have to check your blood from time to time.
- ***Other medications***. If you combine Evista with certain medications you may be more likely to experience side effects. These medications include clofibrate (Atromid-S), a medication used to lower cholesterol levels or to treat diabetes insipidus; indomethacin, naproxen, or ibuprofen, all of which are nonsteroidal anti-inflammatory drugs (NSAIDs)

that relieve pain and inflammation and are sold under a variety of brand names; diazepam, a tranquilizer better known by its brand name Valium; and diazoxide (Hyperstat or Proglycem), a blood-pressure-lowering medication. Taking Evista may also affect people who are taking thyroid medications, so if you are taking this type of medication you should have your blood levels checked before starting on Evista.

Do You Take Any of These Medications? If So, Mention This to Your Doctor Before Starting on Evista

Antibiotics	ampicillin (various brand names)
Estrogen Therapy	ERT or HRT
Blood Thinners	warfarin (Coumadin, Panwarfin, or Sofarin)
Cholesterol-Lowering Medications	clofibrate (Atromid-S) or cholestyramine (Prevalite, Questran, or Questran Light)
Medications That Relieve Pain and Inflammation	indomethacin, naproxen, or ibuprofen, each of which have various brand names
Tranquilizers	diazepam (Valium)
Blood Pressure Medications	diazoxide (Hyperstat or Proglycem)

Q: What is the most serious side effect of Evista?

A: The most serious side effect of Evista is a blood clot in the veins. This side effect is rare and happens more often in women with a history of blood clots. These clots occur in the legs, lungs, or eyes, and are most likely to happen during the first four months of using Evista. Because these clots can prevent blood flow, they can cause serious and chronic problems when they occur—they can even be fatal. It is important to understand the warning signs of a blood clot so that you can get immediate help.

Q: What are some of the common side effects?

A: Most of Evista's side effects are considered mild. The most common side effects associated with Evista are hot flashes and leg cramps. In studies, women who took Evista had a higher rate of hot flashes than did women who took placebos (sugar pills). About 25% of women on Evista experienced hot flashes while only about 18% of women taking placebos had them. Evista does not make your hot flashes feel worse; it simply may cause you to have more of them. It may also cause hot flashes in women who experienced none before starting on the medication. Most women experienced this side effect early on during treatment. After six months on Evista it tended to subside. Women taking Evista also had a higher rate of leg cramps than did women who took placebos (6% versus 2%). As is the case with many medications, including other bone builders, a variety of side effects were reported during the course of the Evista testing that may or may not be caused by the medication itself. Ask your doctor for a full list of Evista's reported side effects.

Warning Signs of a Blood Clot

- Pain in the lower leg or leg swelling
- Sharp chest pain, breathing difficulties, or coughing up of blood
- A sudden change in vision

Q: When I am on Evista, is there anything that I should be careful about?

A: Yes. In order to help avoid getting a blood clot, taking Evista should not coincide with a prolonged period of bed rest, which may happen after surgery or if you are confined to bed due to sickness or injury. If you know that you are going to be confined to bed for a long time—perhaps you are scheduled for surgery—you should always stop taking Evista at least three days (72 hours) before you plan on being laid up. You can go back on Evista again once you are back on your feet.

Even if not confined to bed, it is a good idea to avoid sitting for hours at a time because this also can increase your risk of getting a blood clot. This is especially true during the first four months of using Evista, since that is when blood clots are more likely to occur. When traveling for long periods, it is important to get up and move around every once in awhile. If you are taking a long airplane trip, get up every so often and stretch your legs. During drives to see the grandchildren, remember to take rest stops. A good rule of thumb is to get up and move around every two or three hours or so. Once you get in the habit, it will become second nature. Getting your circulation going has the added benefit of making a monotonously long trip a little more pleasant. If you are bound to a desk all day at work, you should also remember to get up and move around from time to time. Just make sure that you do not take too many coffee breaks—caffeine can reduce the amount of calcium, that all-important building block of bone, absorbed by your body.

6

How to Treat Your Menopausal Symptoms with Alternative and Other Therapies While Taking Evista

Quick Fact: In some women, hot flashes can occur up to a decade after menopause.

Gail was a 53-year-old woman who was seeing me because of severe hot flashes. She had been diagnosed with early breast cancer two years prior and had successfully completed radiation therapy. Three months prior her periods had suddenly ceased and she began to wake up nightly with drenching sweats. The doctor who was treating her breast cancer prescribed tamoxifen (Nolvadex), a selective estrogen receptor modulator (SERM) drug, to treat her cancer, and hormone replacement therapy (HRT) was out of the question. I prescribed a medication called Bellergal (a combination of belladonna and ergotamine with phenobarbital) for Gail, which gave her modest relief, but she still awoke three times a night. When I saw her next she had been through every herbal remedy without relief. Exhausted, she looked for further help. I suggested that she try natural soy estrogens. Many medical studies suggest that a diet high in soy may be the most effective alternative treatment to help to reduce the frequency of hot flashes. I assured Gail that there seemed to be no proven link between natural estrogen and breast cancer, though we could not be 100 percent certain. Gail was willing to try anything and she began taking a soy supplement three times a day. Within a few weeks she called to say that she was nearly sleeping through the night and felt remarkably better at work.

Like many women, you may continue to experience symptoms associated with menopause years after your last menstrual period. You may also encounter new problems during your postmenopausal years that are also related to estrogen loss, such as vaginal dryness and thinning. No one can predict exactly which problems, if any, will affect you the most because they vary from woman to woman. Coping with these symptoms may pose a challenge well after menopause for some women but not for others. Doctors today have a much better understanding of the changes associated with menopause than they ever did. Your doctor knows that the problems you may be facing in the years after menopause are real—not just "in your head"—and has effective treatments. Unfortunately, medical science was not always so enlightened or helpful. Just look at this quote from an 1887 neurological textbook that likens menopause to mental illness:

> The ovaries, after long years of service, have not the ability of retiring in graceful old age, but become irritated, transmit these irritations to the abdominal

> ganglia, which in turn transmit the irritation to the brain producing disturbances in the cerebral tissue exhibiting themselves in extreme nervousness or in an outburst of actual insanity.

Fortunately doctors today know that most of the problems encountered by women during and after menopause—such as hot flashes or night sweats, sleeping difficulties, urinary tract infections (UTIs), vaginal dryness and thinning, moodiness, and forgetfulness—are caused directly or indirectly by the fact that during menopause a woman loses 80% of the estrogen her body once had. The most effective overall treatment for these problems is estrogen replacement therapy (ERT) or hormone replacement therapy (HRT), which replaces the missing estrogen. Evista, on the other hand, does not treat any of these symptoms, and may even cause you to have more hot flashes, at least for the first several months. Since you cannot take ERT or HRT and Evista at the same time, if you choose to make Evista part of your personal strategy to increase the strength of your bones, you will have to find other ways to ease any symptoms that you find troublesome. Other elements of your bone-building strategy will also help you to cope with menopausal symptoms. For example, maintaining a healthy, nutritious diet and exercising regularly actually help to prevent or alleviate some of these symptoms and can improve your mental outlook and reduce stress in the process. There are also a number of specific methods available that treat menopausal symptoms or help to avoid them altogether. These include over-the-counter (OTC) and prescription medications as well as alternative therapies involving herbs and vitamin supplements. Sometimes just learning healthy habits can be enough to alleviate a particular problem.

You probably have heard about some of these alternative

therapies and their exciting claims in the news in recent years. Names like Korean ginseng, ginkgo biloba, and St. John's wort have become familiar to the public, and doctors have gotten serious about investigating these substances in order to confirm what they can and cannot do. The U.S. government has even established an Office of Alternative Medicine in Washington, D.C., to focus on the study of unconventional therapies. As of today, most of these therapies have not been approved by the Food and Drug Administration (FDA) for any purpose. Their safety and effectiveness are largely unregulated by any government agency. But tens of millions of Americans use them and many swear by them. It should be noted, however, that although some of the therapies mentioned in this chapter are in use in European countries such as Germany, European regulation of alternative therapies is not equal to a review by the FDA in terms of efficacy and safety.

Despite the fact that they are often derived from plants, these remedies sometimes have powerful effects that mimic those of natural hormones or prescription medications. For this reason, you should always discuss any of these therapies with a doctor before using them, especially if you are taking Evista or other prescription medication or have existing medical conditions. Forms and recommended dosages can vary, so talk to your doctor or a doctor who has experience with unconventional therapies before you experiment with them. See Chapter 10 for a listing of organizations that can provide more information on alternative therapies and that can help put you in touch with a doctor in your area who prescribes them.

Q: What are hot flashes?

A: About 80% of American women experience hot flashes at some time during menopause, and these hot flashes may continue well after menopause is complete. Hot flashes can be annoying and disruptive. You may get them for months or years. Hot flashes happen when blood vessels near the surface of the skin widen. This is felt as a sudden rush of warmth in the chest that moves up into the neck and face. This hot feeling may spread to other parts of your body as well. Hot flashes can last anywhere from several seconds to several minutes and vary in intensity. During a mild hot flash you may just feel a sensation of warmth that is not very bothersome. In other cases a hot flash may cause your heart to race, you may feel flushed, and you may start to sweat (despite how it feels, there is not usually a change in blood pressure). In some cases you may sweat quite heavily. You may also feel a tingling sensation in your hands. When the hot flash is over your body temperature drops and you may feel chilled. These flashes may occur up to several times a day. They happen most often during the day but can be more intense at night—when they are referred to as ''night sweats''—making it hard to get good, uninterrupted sleep. The worst hot flashes are experienced by women who have had an abrupt loss of ovarian estrogen due to surgery, radiation, or chemotherapy. Because fat helps to convert hormones from the adrenal glands into estrogen, thinner women tend to have less estrogen and as a result have more hot flashes.

Q: What is a hot flash trigger?

A: A trigger in this case is the term used by doctors to describe anything that may set off a hot flash. Possible triggers include hot drinks, spicy foods, hot and humid weather, stress, smoking, marijuana, anger, caffeine, alcohol, and hot rooms or tight, confining spaces such as elevators. By avoiding these common triggers, you may be able to avoid some hot flashes altogether. As you saw in Chapters 1 and 2, smoking, alcohol, and caffeine should be avoided in any case because they each may increase your risk for osteoporosis.

Q: Will I know when a hot flash is about to happen?

A: You certainly may. Some women can actually sense when a hot flash is about to strike. You may simply have a feeling of uneasiness or anxiety—a sense that something is not quite right—that acts as a premonition for what is about to come. Other times you may experience physical symptoms that appear right before a hot flash, such as pressure or pain in your head, nausea, or a tingling sensation. These symptoms, while they may cause you discomfort, act as a warning and give you time to take action before the hot flash is upon you.

Q: What can I do when I sense it coming?

A: While it may not be possible to avoid hot flashes entirely, some forethought and a few commonsense tips may dampen their effects and reduce how often you get them. The way you dress is a good place to start. Be sure to wear natural fibers that breathe, such as cotton or silk. This way some of the heat generated by your body during a flash can escape into the air. It is also important to dress in layers so that you can quickly remove or put on clothing as needed. Drinking a glass of cold water or juice at the start of a hot flash also may help to ease its effects. As strange as it may sound, sucking on a piece of hard candy has been known to help ward off a hot flash.

Q: Can exercise help to ease hot flashes?

A: Yes. Exercise helps to reduce the frequency of hot

Tips for Coping with Hot Flashes or Night Sweats

- Dress in layers so that you can quickly remove or add clothing as needed.
- Avoid triggers.
- Drink a glass of cold water or juice at the start of a hot flash.
- Keep a thermos of ice water by your bed at night for quick relief.
- Wear clothes made with natural fibers (such as cotton or silk) in order to allow your skin to breathe.

flashes by lowering the amount of circulating FSH and FH, hormones made in the pituitary gland that play a role in a woman's reproductive life. Exercise also raises endorphine levels, which drop during a hot flash. About 20 minutes of exercise a day (three or four times a week) can reduce how many hot flashes you experience.

Q: Are there any alternative therapies for hot flashes?

A: In recent years Korean ginseng (*Panax ginseng*) has gained a reputation for helping to alleviate hot flashes. Also known as Chinese ginseng and Ren Shen, Korean ginseng is a small plant that grows in the forests of northeast Asia. It has been used for more than 7,000 years in China for a variety of purposes, and is thought to help ease some typical menopausal symptoms. Some people think that a few capsules of Korean ginseng a day, depending on body weight, can help with hot flashes. Korean ginseng is available in various forms, but capsules are recommended because it is the easiest way to be sure how much Korean ginseng you are getting.

If you take Korean ginseng, it is best to take it on an empty stomach, at least two hours before or after meals. Do not take it at the same time as a vitamin supplement and avoid fruit or fruit juices for a couple of hours after you take it. If you have high blood pressure or diabetes, you may not be able to take Korean ginseng—be sure to talk to your doctor before using it. Korean ginseng may not be a good option for women with emphysema or asthma either, because it may encourage the release of histamine, a chemical released by the body during an allergic reaction. You should also be aware that Korean ginseng has been known to cause mild, short-term breast tenderness.

Some alternative medicine practitioners also recommend vitamin E for hot flashes. It may take several weeks before you know if it is working or not. Vitamin E is found in seeds, nuts, and polyunsaturated vegetable oil and is available over the counter as a supplement. Vitamin E may increase the effects of the blood thinner warfarin (Coumadin, Panwarfin, or Sofarin) or aspirin, so always talk to your doctor before taking vitamin E supplements. Women who are diabetic, have heart conditions, or are taking high blood pressure medication should only take vitamin E under a doctor's supervision.

Black cohosh (*Cimicifuga racemosa*), a plant native to the forests of North America, is another possible remedy for hot flashes. It is also known as squaw root, black snake root, and rattle weed. It was used by American Indians, who used to boil the root and make a sort of tea of it, for a variety of conditions in women. Like

Other Alternative Therapies That May Help to Ease Hot Flashes or Night Sweats

- Bee pollen
- Blue cohosh
- Chickweed tincture
- Dong quai
- False unicorn
- Licorice root
- Motherwort extract
- Primrose oil
- Royal jelly
- Sage tea
- Sarsaparilla
- Wild yam root

certain other alternative approaches, black cohosh has been studied more in Germany, where it is used to treat hot flashes.

Medical studies suggest that a diet high in soy may be the most effective alternative treatment to help to reduce the frequency of hot flashes. Good sources of soy include soy milk, tofu, roasted soy nuts, soy flour, and tempeh. A variety of other alternative therapies, sometimes used in combination, are also used for hot flashes (see chart above).

Q: What if I need something stronger for my hot flashes? Can my doctor prescribe something?

A: Hot flashes do not usually require prescription medication. For many women they simply do not present enough of a problem. But in severe cases your doctor may prescribe a medication such as Bellergal (a combination of belladonna and ergotamine with phenobarbital), which is approved by the FDA to treat hot flashes. One of its ingredients, phenobarbital, can be addicting, so Bellergal should only be used for short periods of time.

Certain medications for blood pressure also have the added benefit of helping to alleviate hot flashes. These medications include clonidine (Catapres), propranolol (Inderal), methyldopa (Aldomet), and medications containing the generic ingredient verapamil (Calan, Covera, Isoptin, or Verelan). Keep in mind that some blood pressure medications have side effects that may make you more likely to fall. As you saw in Chapter 3, a simple fall may be enough to cause a fracture in a woman with osteoporosis.

Q: What are night sweats?

A: Night sweats are hot flashes that occur at night while you are sleeping. Night sweats often wake you from sleep, sometimes several times a night. This can lead to daytime fatigue and can even make you more anxious. Being covered by a blanket or sheet that traps heat may make the effects of night sweats worse. That is why it is important to use natural fibers that breathe, such as cotton or silk, for your covers and bedclothes. Even snuggling with your partner may worsen night sweats because of your partner's body heat. Try opening the windows in your bedroom or running an air conditioner to keep you cool (with your partner's consent!). Keeping a thermos of ice water or an ice pack by your bed at night for quick relief may also help.

Q: Why is it so hard to get a good night's sleep sometimes?

A: Not being able to get continuous and restful sleep is a fairly common complaint during and after menopause. Waking up during the night due to hot flashes is one reason why it may be hard to sleep the whole night through or to sleep well. Once you manage to get these hot flashes under control or to ease their effects, you will probably find it much easier to get restful, uninterrupted sleep. Loss of estrogen may affect the quality of your sleep in other ways as well by interfering with deep REM sleep. As a result of this interference, you may not feel as refreshed and rejuvenated during the day as you should.

Q: What is sleep hygiene?

A: *Sleep hygiene* is simply a phrase used to describe behavioral habits that may help or hurt how well you sleep. As everyone knows, practicing good *dental* hygiene helps to keep your teeth cavity free. Practicing good sleep hygiene helps you to fall or stay asleep, often by avoiding bad sleep habits (which you may not even know that you have). Here are some tips to help you fall asleep faster and improve the quality of your sleep:

- ***Go to bed and wake up about the same time each day***. Despite what you may believe, it is actually counterproductive to try and make up for lack of sleep on weekends, holidays, or days off from work. A regular sleep schedule is the best approach.

Taking frequent naps during the day is also not recommended.

- ***Avoid conflict.*** In the several hours before you go to bed, try to avoid arguments or other things that involve negative emotions. Do not focus on problems or things that are bothering you. Do something that you find relaxing instead, such as taking a bath.
- ***Relax your muscles***. Try a relaxation exercise, such as tensing and relaxing different muscle groups. Start with your toes and end with your neck and shoulder muscles. Ask your doctor about other relaxation exercises.
- ***Limit your activities in the bedroom***. Your bedroom should only be a place for sleep and sex. Do not watch TV, pay bills, or do other activities in your bedroom.
- ***If you cannot sleep, get up***. If you are having trouble falling asleep, do not spend a long time lying awake in bed. Get up and do something else in another room until you feel sleepier, such as watching TV or reading a book.
- ***Avoid caffeine and alcohol***. Do not drink caffeine or alcohol during the several hours before you go to sleep. You probably thought that alcohol *helps* people sleep. That is partly true. A glass of wine in the evening may in fact help you fall asleep faster. But too much alcohol, while it may put you to sleep fairly quickly, disrupts the quality of your sleep as the night wears on. You should also be aware that many OTC medications—including some allergy, decongestant, cold remedy, and painkilling medications—contain caffeine.
- ***Be active.*** Exercise during the day or in the early evening may make it easier to sleep, but do not

exercise in the three hours before you go to bed, or the exercise may actually make it harder to doze off. Stay busy enough during the day so that you are tired at night.

Q: What else can I do to help me sleep?

A: In addition to the OTC sleep aids in your local pharmacy, there are several alternative remedies that may help. The first of these is called kava (*Piper methysticum*). Also known as kava kava or kawa, this Polynesian shrub (a member of the pepper family) was known as the "intoxicating pepper" in times past and is now used worldwide for sleeplessness and to curb anxiety. Unlike most remedies for sleeplessness, kava does not get less effective over time, according to its proponents. If you are taking a prescription antidepressant medication, you may not be able to take kava. Another possible sleep aid is valerian root (*Valeriana officinalis*), also called Capon's tail or English valerian. This herb is native to Europe and was used in ancient Rome as a mild sedative. Like kava, it is used to help people sleep and to relieve anxiety. Some medical studies suggest that valerian root may help to ease occasional insomnia.

Prescription medications are available as well. In some cases your doctor may prescribe sleeping pills such as zolpidem (Ambien) or temazepam (Restoril) for short periods of time. Although not strongly physically addicting in the long term, habituation and dependence can occur. If your sleeping difficulties continue despite treatment, you and your doctor will need to investigate the underlying cause more thoroughly. Depression and anxiety are the most common causes of chronic sleeping problems, though in up to 30% of cases no cause can be identified.

Q: Can I do anything for the fatigue that I feel during the day?

A: Your fatigue may simply be due to the fact that you are not getting a good night's rest, in which case some of the remedies for night sweats or sleeplessness discussed earlier in the chapter may help. Some women who have completed menopause report feeling fatigue even in the absence of any sleeping difficulties. Whatever the reason for the fatigue, Korean ginseng may be what you need to put a little more pep in your step. As an added benefit, Korean ginseng may be able to help prevent thinning of the vagina, which can make sex uncomfortable.

Q: I seem to get more UTIs these days than I ever did before. Why is that?

A: During and after menopause, women are more vulnerable to these sometimes painful infections. This is because as your body loses estrogen, the tissues of the urinary tract become thinner and are more easily irritated. A urinary infection happens when a part of your urinary tract is invaded by large numbers of bacteria. Usually the bacterium *Escherichia coli* is the culprit. This infection can occur in the urethra (the tube leading from the bladder to the outside of the body), the bladder, or the kidneys. Women tend to get UTIs more often than do men because the short length of the urethra in women allows bacteria into the bladder more easily. The symptoms of a urinary tract infection include a burning sensation when urinating, an urgent need to urinate, and frequent urination. Once a UTI occurs, it can be treated effectively by your doctor with antibiotics.

Q: Can anything be done to prevent UTIs?

A: Although you may not be able to avoid UTIs altogether,

Things You Can Do to Help Avoid UTIs

- After a bowel movement, always wipe upward from front to back.
- Urinate before and after sex.
- Drink 10 ounces of cranberry juice a day.
- Drink 6 to 8 glasses of water throughout the day (6-ounce glasses).
- Avoid possible irritants such as bubble bath solution or the chlorine used in swimming pools.

medical studies suggest that you can reduce your risk of getting them simply by drinking about 10 ounces of cranberry juice every day. Echinacea (*Echinacea augustifolia*) is another possibility. Also called purple coneflower, this herb native to the American Midwest was widely used by Native Americans. Medical studies in Germany suggest that echinacea may be able to strengthen the immune system. It may be helpful in heading off urinary infections in women who get them often. You may also be able to lessen your risk of a UTI by learning some healthy habits (see the chart above).

Q: Am I the only woman who finds sex uncomfortable after menopause?

A: No, you are definitely not alone, and the good news is that it is not something that you have to live with. Many women find sex a little uncomfortable to some degree after menopause. This is because the walls of the vagina become thinner, dryer, and less elastic as your body loses estrogen. The outer lips of the vagina shrink, and the vagina itself becomes shorter or narrower. As was mentioned earlier, these tissues also become more sensitive to irritation, and this may make sex more uncomfortable, even painful.

It is important to understand that vaginal dryness or thinning is a physical problem. It is different from sexual desire or libido, though naturally your sexual desire may be affected to some degree when sex becomes physically uncomfortable. Many factors can affect the nature of your sexual desire—including stress, depression, and being angry with your partner—and these underlying reasons cannot be addressed by the remedies described here. If you are concerned about a possible loss of sex drive, talk to your doctor.

Q: What can I do to make sex pain-free and enjoyable again?

A: The most effective treatment for vaginal dryness and thinning is ERT or HRT, which you cannot use if you are taking Evista. But even if you are on Evista, you can use the next best thing, a prescription estrogen cream (inserted into the vagina once a week), for a short period of time if your doctor thinks that it is justified. For women with a mild problem, water-based vaginal lubricants, many of which are available over the counter, can help to relieve vaginal dryness and pain during intercourse. Some of these lubricants also have the added benefit of helping to reduce the risk of infections. In addition to these methods, regular sexual intercourse or stimulation will also combat dryness naturally by generating vaginal secretions.

There are two alternative therapies that may also help.

The first is Korean ginseng, which some studies suggest may help to prevent thinning of the vagina. The second is goldenseal (*Hydrastis canadensis*), a small North American plant with a single red fruit once used by Native Americans for local infections or inflammation. Some alternative medicine practitioners believe that it is useful for vaginal irritation and inflammation in women who have completed menopause. Its other names include Seal-all, golden thread, yellow root, and Indian dye.

Q: Sometimes I catch myself feeling anxious or moody. It really is not like me to feel this way but I cannot help it. Is this normal?

A: With all the changes that go on during and after menopause, it is no wonder that so many women experience emotions like these. Between 30% to 70% of postmenopausal women complain of symptoms such as moodiness, crying, anxiety, and irritability. Although some of these feelings are probably a result of low estrogen levels, the challenge of adjusting to a new and important stage in life can also have an effect on your emotions. Women who do not approach menopause in a positive way or who lack the support and understanding of friends and loved ones tend to have a harder time making the adjustment. The negative emotions that some women have during and after menopause may also reflect their fears of getting older or feeling less attractive.

Some women also suffer depression in their menopausal years. Twenty-five percent of women develop some form of depression in their lifetimes. Depression is not the same thing as feeling occasionally moody or having a mild case of the blues. It is a serious, sometimes life-threatening medical condition that requires a doctor's care. If you think you are suffering from depression, talk to your doctor right away. There is no need to suffer from this debilitating condition alone. Your doctor has many effective ways to treat depression and help you feel like your old self again.

Q: Are there any alternative remedies that I can use to alleviate moodiness or anxiety?

A: Do not forget about regular exercise, which can improve mood and help take the edge off anxiety. Several alternative therapies make claims to soothe the nerves or give the spirit a boost. The most well known of these is probably St. John's wort (*Hypericum perforatum*). This plant, found in Europe and the United States, was used during the Middle Ages for anxiety and depression, among other things. In Germany it is approved by the government for the treatment of mild depression, where it has been prescribed by doctors in literally millions of cases. St. John's wort has powerful effects, some of which mimic those of the prescription antidepressant medication Prozac. You should always talk to your doctor first before using this popular remedy, which must be taken for several weeks before its effects are felt. St. John's wort may not be taken along with prescription antidepressants. If you take St. John's wort, you should avoid certain foods and beverages such as aged cheese, beer, and wine. In addition to St. John's wort, kava and valerian root are used by some women to ease anxiety as well as sleeplessness. Several German medical studies suggest that kava is safe and may help to relieve anxiety as well as certain prescription medications. If you are taking a prescription antidepressant medication, you may not be able to take kava. Some women also find that meditation can also be useful in curbing anxiety or moodiness.

Warning Signs of Depression

Talk to your doctor if you have had four or more of the following symptoms for more than two weeks.

- Changes in appetite, with either significant weight loss (that is not due to dieting) or weight gain
- Changes in sleeping patterns, such as fitful sleep, inability to sleep, early morning awakening, or sleeping too much
- Loss of interest or pleasure in activities that you once enjoyed
- Fatigue or loss of energy
- Feelings of worthlessness
- Constant feelings of hopelessness
- Feelings of inappropriate guilt
- Indecisiveness or an inability to concentrate or think
- Repeated thoughts of death or suicide, a wish to die, or a suicide attempt (Note: People with this symptom should seek treatment immediately.)
- Overwhelming feelings of sadness or grief accompanied by waking at least two hours earlier than normal in the morning, feeling more depressed in the morning, and moving significantly more slowly
- Disturbed thinking
- Physical symptoms such as headache or stomachache

Source: Adapted with permission from the *Diagnostic and Statistical Manual of Mental Disorders, Fourth Edition*. Copyright 1994 American Psychiatric Association.

Q: As someone who has been known to misplace her car keys from time to time, I know my memory is not perfect. But I seem to be forgetting a lot of little things lately that I never used to. Is this just my imagination?

A: Probably not. This memory loss or forgetfulness is often due to a decline in estrogen levels. It is a fairly common complaint of women who have completed menopause, either naturally or due to surgery. Estrogen therapy has been shown in medical studies to actually enhance memory. If you are taking Evista and are bothered by the feeling that you are forgetting things, you may wish to try ginkgo biloba (*Ginkgo biloba*). This species of plant, also called maidenhair tree and bai guo, has been used for more than 5,000 years in China, mainly for breathing difficulties and for its beneficial effects on the brain, and it is thought to be useful for forgetfulness in postmenopausal women.

Some women use ginkgo biloba in combination with hawthorn (*Crataegus oxyacantha*) for forgetfulness. Hawthorn, a European tree with bright red berries, has been used since the Middle Ages and is thought to widen blood vessels and improve circulation. Also called mayflower, may bush, and English hawthorn, hawthorn has been used in China, Europe, and America for heart and circulatory disorders. So far there is no evidence to suggest that ginkgo biloba is more effective when combined with hawthorn than it is when used alone.

Q: Is Alzheimer's disease just a bad case of being forgetful?

A: No. Alzheimer's is a serious and debilitating medical condition that gets progressively worse over time (usually over a period of six to eight years) and is eventually fatal. Its exact causes are unknown (family history seems to play a role), and there is no cure. An estimated 4 million Americans now have Alzheimer's. Three times as many women get it as men and more than 90% of cases are found in people over age 65. In early stages of the disease, people with Alzheimer's suffer from memory loss and confusion. A person with Alzheimer's may get lost even in familiar surroundings and have problems doing everyday tasks. Later there are changes in personality and judgment. Anxiety and sleeping difficulties worsen. A person with Alzheimer's may even have trouble with feeding and bathing. In the last stages, a person with Alzheimer's has trouble speaking, cannot recognize friends and loved ones, and becomes totally dependent on others.

Q: Is there anything that I can take to help prevent Alzheimer's?

A: Estrogen therapy is the only medication that potentially may help to prevent or delay development of Alzheimer's in women. Medical studies suggest that ERT and HRT can greatly improve functioning in women with Alzheimer's, and postmenopausal women who receive ERT or HRT are 40% to 60% less likely to develop the disease in the first place. There are also two medications approved by the FDA for the treatment of Alzheimer's—tacrine (Cognex) and donepezil (Aricept)—but these medications do not prevent it. They only provide temporary improvement in some cases of mild or moderate Alzheimer's.

Q: Are there any alternative approaches to preventing Alzheimer's?

A: There are some new alternative approaches being studied, involving ginkgo biloba and vitamin E, but the jury is still out as to whether or not they are effective at preventing the condition. Ginkgo biloba has recently been approved in Germany for the treatment of Alzheimer's. A 1997 study in the *Journal of the American Medical Association*, a medical journal, suggests that ginkgo biloba can stabilize and improve mental performance and social functioning for six months to one year in people with Alzheimer's. In another 1997 study published in the *New England Journal of Medicine*, vitamin E appeared to slow the progression of the disease. Vitamin E is found in seeds, nuts, and polyunsaturated vegetable oil and is available over the counter as a supplement. Vitamin E may increase the effects of the blood thinner warfarin (Coumadin, Panwarfin, or Sofarin) or aspirin, so always talk to your doctor before taking regular vitamin E supplements. Women who are diabetic, have heart conditions, or are taking high blood pressure medication should take vitamin E only under a doctor's supervision. As of early 1999, it was not clear if taking ginkgo biloba or vitamin E supplements would help to prevent the onset of Alzheimer's. Talk to your doctor about the latest scientific thinking on these approaches.

7

Other Medications Used to Prevent or Treat Osteoporosis

Quick Fact: Estrogen therapy may reduce your risk of heart attack by up to 50%.

Brenda is a longstanding patient of mine. Despite my best efforts at counseling, she smoked two packs of cigarettes a day for 25 years. At age 52, she began hormone replacement therapy (HRT), but after three months on therapy she developed a blood clot in her left leg. Smoking had put her more at risk for blood clots. Although she stopped smoking, she was now quite concerned about her health. An exercise stress test indicated no problems in the cardiovascular area, but Brenda's bone density score was 2.5, which indicates the presence of osteoporosis (her smoking was a contributing factor). HRT and Evista were both ruled out as options because of the blood clot. Brenda wanted to know more about alendronate (Fosamax) and the hormone calcitonin. I explained the side effects of each, and Brenda decided to use the strongest bone builder, alendronate.

Before deciding whether or not to make Evista the focus of your personalized bone-building strategy, you and your doctor will need to weigh the advantages and disadvantages of the three other osteoporosis medications approved by the Food and Drug Administration (FDA). Like Evista, each of these medications must be used regularly for a period of years, and in some cases decades, in order to maintain healthy bones. The most commonly prescribed medication for osteoporosis is estrogen replacement therapy (ERT), known as hormone replacement therapy (HRT) when combined with the hormone progesterone. Estrogen has been studied by doctors for decades and is often referred to as the gold standard, the measurement by which all other menopausal therapies are judged. It has earned this distinction because of its wide-ranging, healthy effects on various menopausal symptoms (such as hot flashes and vaginal dryness and thinning) and on serious conditions that women are more vulnerable to as they age, including osteoporosis, heart disease, and Alzheimer's disease. Despite the proven health benefits of ERT and HRT, only about 20% of the 40 million postmenopausal women in the United States end up choosing this type of therapy. Some are afraid that it may increase the risk of cancer while others find the side effects bothersome.

The most powerful bone builder of all is alendronate (Fosamax). Approved for the prevention and treatment of osteoporosis in the mid-1990s, this nonhormonal medication has an unequaled effect when it comes to increasing bone density in the hip, spine, or wrist—where most women with osteoporosis tend to fracture bones. Alendronate is strictly a therapy for osteoporosis. You cannot use it to ease your menopausal symptoms and it does not confer any protective effects on the heart or brain as do ERT and HRT. Calcitonin (Calcimar or Miacalcin) came on the market around the same time as alendronate. Commonly used in the newer nasal spray form (Miacalcin), calcitonin is only used in women with existing osteoporosis who have not had a menstrual period in at least five years. Calcitonin is primarily used to increase bone density in the spine and is not considered to be very useful in making bones stronger in the hip or wrist. Like alendronate, calcitonin cannot be used for any purpose other than increasing bone density. Both alendronate and calcitonin are usually considered options for women who cannot or choose not to use ERT or HRT.

You may be thinking, "Why not take two or more of these medications in order to get the best combination of possible effects?" Doctors have asked themselves the same question. Research is now going on to find out if alendronate and estrogen can be combined as part of a "best of both worlds" approach. But as of early 1999 the safety of taking any of these medications together had not been established and in some cases could be dangerous. For now, you and your doctor must evaluate each therapy on its own merits, in light of your medical history and your health goals and concerns. For example, women who take alendronate or calcitonin must find other ways to cope with menopausal symptoms and to protect themselves against the potentially deadly consequences of heart disease. Women with a family history of breast cancer might be inclined to choose Evista over ERT or HRT, while women who are at high risk for blood clots may find that alendronate or calcitonin is the safest option for them. It is a decision that must be made carefully when you consider that every available osteoporosis medication must be taken regularly for a period of at least several years. In addition to medication, your personal strategy for preventing or treating osteoporosis will also include calcium and vitamin D supplements when appropriate and you should continue to follow the diet and exercise regimen prescribed by your doctor.

Q: What is estrogen therapy?

A: Estrogen therapy is as close as medical science has come to finding a single medication that meets the various challenges to health and well-being posed by the loss of estrogen due to menopause. Estrogen, which has been used and studied for decades longer than any other osteoporosis medication, can be used to ease the symptoms of menopause as well as to prevent serious conditions affecting the bones, heart, and brain. Estrogen is an effective bone-building medication that can increase bone density by about 4% to 5% on average. When used during or after menopause it can delay or prevent the weakening of bones. In fact, if you are on ERT or HRT, there is an 85% chance that you will prevent bone loss. In addition to increasing bone density, ERT and HRT have also been shown to reduce the risk of fractures. Studies show that women on ERT or HRT have about half as many hip fractures—the most serious type of fracture—as those who do not take it. Estrogen also reduces the risk of wrist fractures and compression fractures in the spine. It is used to help prevent heart disease and may prevent the risk of heart attack by up to 50%. Recent research also indicates that estrogen may reduce the risk of Alzheimer's disease, a serious and debilitating condition affecting the functioning of the brain, by 50%. See Chapter 6 for more information about Alzheimer's and the use of estrogen to help prevent it.

Q: How is estrogen therapy different from Evista?

A: ERT and HRT work by replacing the estrogen that your

Why Women Take Estrogen

- To prevent osteoporosis
- To prevent heart disease
- To control menopausal symptoms
- To maintain sexual function
- To prevent Alzheimer's disease

body loses during menopause with a version of the hormone made in a laboratory. Although Evista is also a hormonal medication, estrogen therapy is different than Evista both in terms of its chemistry and its effects on your health. Evista and other SERMs are chemical copycats. They are designed to act like estrogen in some parts of the body and to block the effects of estrogen in other parts. Estrogen therapy, on the other hand, is a way of restoring the estrogen that your body has lost. It does not make decisions about when to act like estrogen and when not to.

Q: How do I take estrogen?

A: Estrogen is available as a pill, patch, or cream. Pills with the brand name Premarin are the most commonly prescribed form of estrogen in the United States. Premarin contains conjugated equine estrogens, which are really several forms of estrogen taken from the urine of pregnant mares. In order to get the full benefits of estrogen therapy, you must use the pill or patch form. Like Evista, estrogen therapy must be taken regularly in order to be effective. Once you stop using it you lose its protective effects. The patch, which contains a purer form of estrogen called estradiol, can be placed anywhere on the upper body, including the abdomen or buttocks, but not on the breasts. In the past estrogen patches were usually used on a schedule of three weeks on, one week off, though in some cases an estrogen patch could be worn all the time without a break. We now know that this schedule of alternated doses diminishes estrogen's protective effects and estrogen is now given continuously without a break. Estrogen cream is primarily used to treat drying and thinning of the vagina that occurs due to estrogen loss. As you saw in Chapter 6, changes to the vagina during and after menopause can make sex uncomfortable for some women, and estrogen (whether in pill, patch, or cream form) is very effective in alleviating this problem. If you use the cream, only small amounts of estrogen enter your bloodstream. For this reason, the cream does not have any significant benefits on the bones or the heart and it will not ease most menopausal symptoms. It is usually reserved for women who cannot or choose not to take standard estrogen therapy.

Q: What is progesterone?

A: Like estrogen, progesterone is a female sex hormone made by your ovaries until menopause. It is closely involved in your reproductive life and health and is primarily responsible for preparing the uterus for the fertilized egg and for the growth and development of the fetus. Progesterone, usually in a synthetic form called medroxyprogesterone (sold under various brand names), is added to estrogen therapy in order to prevent uterine cancer. While estrogen alone has been shown to greatly increase the risk of this type of cancer, the combination of progesterone and estrogen sharply reduces that risk.

There are disadvantages associated with HRT as well. For one thing, some women experience monthly, menstrual-type bleeding on certain HRT regimens, though this bleeding may cease over a period of years as your uterus ages. Using continuous rather than cyclical doses of progesterone may make vaginal bleeding less likely. HRT taken continuously eliminates vaginal bleeding after a few months, and women can get the benefit of HRT without menstrual bleeding. In addition to menstrual-type bleeding, progesterone can also cause breast tenderness and temporary bloating and in higher doses may dampen your mood or cause you to feel down. Perhaps most importantly, progesterone can slightly reduce estrogen's healthy effects on the heart.

Q: Does estrogen help with hot flashes and other menopausal symptoms?

A: Yes, in a significant way. ERT and HRT have a positive effect on a variety of menopausal symptoms. Estrogen therapy is very effective in alleviating hot flashes, those sudden rushes of warmth in the chest, face, and neck that can last anywhere from several seconds to several minutes. About 80% of menopausal women experience hot flashes, and some women even continue to have hot flashes up to a decade after menopause is complete. As you might expect, estrogen is also very effective in treating night sweats, which are basically hot flashes that occur at night, disrupting sleep and resulting in daytime fatigue and anxiety. Estrogen also helps to reverse some of the changes that occur in your vagina due to estrogen loss. As you saw in Chapter 6, when the body loses estrogen the walls of the vagina become thinner, dryer, and less elastic. The outer lips of the vagina shrink, and the vagina itself becomes shorter or narrower. These tissues become more sensitive to irritation, and this may make sex uncomfortable. ERT and HRT can thicken the vaginal walls, make them more elastic, and signal the vagina to produce more lubrication, all of which helps to ease discomfort. Estrogen therapy also makes urinary tract infections less likely. Estrogen can affect the way that you feel. It appears to alleviate some of the moodiness and anxiety that many menopausal women complain of. But it may also make depression worse in women who are already suffering from non-menopause–related depression. The progesterone therapy taken as a part of HRT may also worsen some symptoms of depression. Estrogen, especially when given with testosterone, may have a welcome effect on your skin, making it look younger, more supple, and thicker.

Q: How does estrogen therapy help prevent heart disease?

A: Protection from heart disease is important if you are a postmenopausal woman. Your risk of heart attack rises steadily after menopause is complete, and in about six to ten years actually equals that of men. Many doctors think that estrogen is the main protective factor against heart disease, which is probably why a woman's risk increases as her body loses estrogen during menopause. The risk rises even faster in the case of surgically induced menopause. Estrogen therapy has a healthy effect on the cardiovascular system and reduces the risk of heart attack. It does this in part by affecting cholesterol levels. ERT and HRT increase levels of high-density lipoprotein (HDL)—the so-called "good" cholesterol—and lower levels of low density lipoprotein (LDL)—the so-called "bad" cholesterol. Raising HDL levels is important. According to the American Heart Association

(AHA), even a small increase in HDL levels can reduce the risk of heart disease by 25%. The major protective effect of estrogen appears to be helping blood vessels relax and increasing blood flow in response to exercise and stress, and keeping blood vessels healthy. Studies support the idea that estrogen has a healthy effect on cholesterol levels and can reduce the risk of death due to heart disease. In the Nurses Health Study, a major trial involving more than 48,000 women who were followed for ten years, the risk of heart attack was cut by almost 50% in women who took estrogen as compared to those who did not. Other studies have shown that ERT and HRT can reduce the risk of heart attack by 30% to 50%. In another important study, the three-year Postmenopausal Estrogen/Progestin Intervention (PEPI) Trial, ERT and HRT were found to significantly increase HDL levels. Because progesterone can slightly reduce the healthy effect of estrogen on the heart, ERT tends to increase HDL levels more than does HRT.

Q: What are androgens and can they really spice up my sex life?

A: Androgens are male sex hormones. You may be surprised to learn that a woman's body also produces these hormones, but in much smaller amounts than in men. Before menopause, androgens (mostly testosterone) are produced by the ovaries and adrenal glands. After menopause is complete, the ovaries stop making androgens. Some androgens are still produced by the adrenal glands but in much smaller amounts. Androgens can be added to estrogen therapy with interesting results. Combined estrogen-androgen therapy (Estratest) may help to improve mood and energy levels, and make your skin look and feel better. Several studies suggest that androgens can also help to improve sex drive in postmenopausal women. In one study of 136 postmenopausal women who complained of sexual problems—termed *sexual dysfunction* by doctors—80% of the women who received the estrogen-androgen combination therapy reported an improvement in libido. Estrogen therapy alone can relieve the vaginal dryness and thinning that causes uncomfortable sex but does not appear to actually increase sex drive.

Androgens have disadvantages as well that must be weighed against their possible benefits. They can cause virilization, a medical term for the development of masculine sex characteristics such as a deepening voice, acne, hair loss, and increased muscle mass. They may also cause the appearance of facial hair, a condition called *hirsuitism*. But these side effects of androgens are usually mild and can be reversed by stopping the androgen part of the therapy or experimenting with a lower dosage. Some studies even show that women on androgens experience fewer of these problems, so we will have to wait for more research in order to get the full picture. Unfortunately, estrogen-androgen therapy has also been shown to decrease HDL levels. This is important because, as you saw earlier in this chapter, higher HDL levels have a protective effect against heart disease and may reduce your risk of heart attack. You should be sure to discuss this effect of androgens with your doctor if you are interested in estrogen-androgen therapy. You may be able to use it for a short period of time and then go back to estrogen therapy without androgens. The long-term risks of estrogen-androgen therapy are also not well understood and more testing is necessary.

Q: Can estrogen therapy cause cancer of the breast or uterus?

A: This is an important question for every woman who considers ERT or HRT, and unfortunately, doctors do not yet have all the answers. First let us talk about what we do know. It is well established that estrogen therapy alone greatly increases the risk of cancer of the uterus by encouraging the growth of cancerous cells. In a woman who has had her uterus removed due to a hysterectomy, this does not present a problem. But in a woman with an intact uterus, HRT is recommended. Doctors generally agree that HRT does not appear to increase the risk of cancer of the uterus.

The jury is still out on the controversial issue of whether or not ERT and HRT can increase your risk for breast cancer. In some studies estrogen therapy has not been linked with any increase in breast cancer, but other studies suggest that the risk of breast cancer may increase with its use. This increased risk is linked to women who have used ERT or HRT for ten years. The truth is that doctors simply do not agree on whether or not ERT and HRT poses a genuine breast cancer threat. Until doctors have resolved this issue, the best course is probably to assume that it does pose some risk. If you have a family history of breast cancer or are particularly concerned about it, estrogen therapy may not be the right choice for you.

Q: What are the side effects of using estrogen therapy?

A: Estrogen and progesterone have different side effects. Women on ERT will have only estrogen-related side effects, whereas women on HRT are susceptible to both. Breast tenderness or enlargement, menstrual-type bleeding or spotting, and weight gain are some of the complaints of women on estrogen therapy. Other side effects include swelling in the ankle or leg, appetite loss, nausea or vomiting, cramps, or a feeling of bloatedness. Estrogen therapy also has the potential to cause more serious problems. It may increase the risk of gallbladder disease in postmenopausal women by two to three times. Like Evista, estrogen therapy may also increase your risk of a blood clot. Because these clots can prevent blood flow, they can cause serious and chronic problems when they occur; they can even be fatal. Women who are on estrogen therapy for long periods of time may also be at risk for blood-clotting disorders, liver cancer or other liver problems, or increased blood pressure. Women who use vaginal estrogen cream do not usually experience any of the side effects described above because very little estrogen actually enters the bloodstream when used in this way, but some women who use the cream experience vaginal bleeding, breast tenderness, or vaginal discharge.

Q: How does Evista compare to estrogen therapy?

A: Both Evista and ERT or HRT are therapies that must be taken regularly for a period of years or even decades in order to be effective. Once you stop taking Evista or estrogen therapy, you lose the protective effect of the medication. Both Evista and estrogen therapy appear to offer other health benefits in addition to making bones healthier. Here is how Evista and estrogen therapy stack up to each other in some key areas.

- ***Osteoporosis.*** Both medications help to prevent bone loss and to increase bone density. ERT and HRT have a slight edge over Evista in that they tend to increase bone density more. Evista causes increases of about 2% to 4% while estrogen therapy tends to increase density by about 4% to 5%. Estrogen therapy has been shown to reduce the risk

A Sampling of Side Effects: Percentage of Women Who Experienced Side Effects on Evista Versus Those Who Took Estrogen

Side Effect	Evista	HRT (continuous combined)	HRT (cyclic)
Breast pain	4.4%	37.5%	29.7%
Vaginal bleeding	6.2%	64.2%	88.5%
Gas	1.6%	12.5%	6.4%
Hot flashes	28.7%	3.1%	5.9%
Stomach pain	6.6%	10.4%	18.7%
Chest pain	2.8%	0%	0.5%

of fractures due to weakened bones. It may cut your risk of hip fracture in half and also make wrist fractures and compression fractures of the spine less likely. Because Evista is a new medication, there have been no studies that show whether or not it will actually reduce your risk of fracturing a bone due to low bone density. Most doctors think that it will, because increasing bone density usually helps to prevent fractures. Studies are now under way to find out in a more direct way if women using Evista are less likely to suffer fractures.

- ***Heart disease.*** Cardiovascular disease is the most common cause of death in women over age 50. Both Evista and estrogen therapy appear to have a protective effect on the heart. Studies suggest that Evista reduces total blood cholesterol levels and LDL levels. This suggests that Evista may help to prevent heart disease. It does not appear to increase levels of HDL. Estrogen therapy, on the other hand, increases HDL levels *and* lowers LDL levels, so it may be more effective in preventing heart disease than is Evista. Studies suggest that ERT and HRT can reduce the risk of heart attack by 30% to 50%. Studies are ongoing to determine whether Evista can reduce the number of heart attacks in postmenopausal women. Evista's possible protective effects on the heart have not been approved by the FDA. It is likely that Evista will be approved by the FDA for preventing heart disease in the next several years.

- ***Menopausal symptoms.*** ERT and HRT are effective in alleviating a wide range of menopausal symptoms, from hot flashes to vaginal dryness and thinning. Estrogen-androgen therapy appears to increase sex drive in some postmenopausal women. Unlike estrogen therapy, Evista does nothing to alleviate menopausal symptoms and may even increase the number of hot flashes you experience or cause you to have them even if you had not had them before, at least for the first six months or so of use. If you choose to use Evista and are bothered by menopausal symptoms, you will have to use means other than ERT or HRT to treat them. See Chapter 6 for more information on how to treat menopausal symptoms while taking Evista.
- ***Cancer of the breast or uterus.*** Despite the fact that estrogen therapy offers a variety of benefits for women after menopause—from easing hot flashes

and vaginal dryness to preventing osteoporosis and heart disease—20% of postmenopausal women actually take estrogen. This is due in part to fears that its effects on the breast and uterus will lead to cancer. After two and a half years of study, Evista does not appear to increase the risk of cancer in the uterus or breast. In fact, studies suggest that Evista may offer protection against breast cancer in postmenopausal women, making it the only other medication besides tamoxifen (Nolvadex) thought to possibly have a protective effect against this disease.

- ***Alzheimer's disease.*** Recent research suggests that estrogen therapy may cut the risk of Alzheimer's and certainly improves mood and performance states in healthy women. Evista, on the other hand, does not appear to have any effect on brain functioning. See Chapter 6 for more information on the debilitating effects of Alzheimer's.

Q: Which osteoporosis medication strengthens bones the most?

A: Alendronate takes the prize as the best bone builder. This medication, belonging to the bisphosphonate class, is the only nonhormonal osteoporosis medication. It cannot be used to treat menopausal symptoms and does not appear to have a healthy effect on the heart or on other parts of the body. But it has been shown to increase bone density more than any other medication, including Evista and estrogen therapy. It may only be used by women who have completed menopause, and it works by slowing down the activity of the bone cells called osteoclasts. Osteoclasts are the biological wrecking crew of cells whose job it is to break down and remove bits of bone.

By putting the brakes on the activities of these cells, alendronate allows other bone cells called osteoblasts—these are the construction worker cells—to build new bone faster than the osteoclasts can destroy old bone. Alendronate is often used in women who cannot or choose not to take ERT or HRT, though doctors are studying the safety and effectiveness of taking alendronate and estrogen therapy together.

Alendronate was approved by the FDA in 1995. In order to gain approval, it was studied in 1,827 postmenopausal women with osteoporosis in 16 countries. In these studies, alendronate was able to increase bone density by 8.2% in the spine and 7.2% in the hip. It was also shown to increase bone strength at other sites. Research suggests that alendronate may cut the risk of spinal fractures by almost 50%. Most side effects were reported as mild; however, because of the somewhat inconvenient method of taking alendronate and stomach upset, some women found the medication difficult to tolerate. Common side effects include stomach pain, upset stomach, nausea, heartburn, diarrhea, stomach gas, and irritation or pain in the esophagus. Women who use alendronate have to be careful about how they take it. Taking it the wrong way can make it less effective and can increase the risk of sometimes dangerous side effects. For example, alendronate is usually taken each morning with a glass of water before having anything to eat or drink and before taking any other medication. It is important to wait at least 30 minutes after taking alendronate before eating or taking other medication in order to make sure that the medication is properly absorbed by the body. The less of the medication that is absorbed, the less well it will work to make your bones stronger. It is also important not to lie down for at least 30 minutes after you take alendronate. It can irritate (or even damage) the esophagus or cause heartburn if you lie down right after taking it.

Q: What is calcitonin?

A: Calcitonin is a hormone found in the human body and in about a dozen other forms of life, including fish. In people, it is produced by the thyroid gland and helps to control how much calcium—that all-important building block of bone—is removed by osteoclasts and sent back into the bloodstream. Like alendronate, calcitonin is only used for osteoporosis and does not have any effect on menopausal symptoms or have other health benefits (though calcitonin may also help to relieve pain due to compression fractures in the spine). It was approved by the FDA in 1995 for the treatment of existing osteoporosis but has not been approved for preventing the condition. The type of calcitonin used to treat osteoporosis is called salmon calcitonin. The name is misleading because it does not come from fish. It is a synthetic form of calcitonin designed to resemble that found in salmon.

Like alendronate, calcitonin helps to prevent bone loss by slowing down the activity of bone-destroying osteoclast cells. Calcitonin, taken daily, is most effective in preventing bone loss in the spine. It does not appear to have lasting bone-building effects in the hip or wrist. The jury is also out on whether or not calcitonin is effective in reducing the risk of fracture, which is the main goal of any osteoporosis therapy. Calcitonin is available as an injection (Calcimar), but most women choose the nasal spray form (Miacalcin). It is for use in women five years after menopause and is usually recommended for women who cannot or choose not to take estrogen therapy. Common side effects include nasal irritation and nasal dryness, redness, itching, or bleeding.

Q: Are there other medications being studied for osteoporosis?

A: Plenty. In addition to other selective estrogen receptor modulators (SERMs), there are a variety of medications on the horizon for preventing or treating osteoporosis. These medications are listed below. See Chapter 9 for more information on the future of SERMs in the treatment of osteoporosis and other conditions.

- ***Bisphosphonates***. Etidronate (Didronel), already approved by the FDA for Paget's disease of the bone, and other chemical cousins of alendronate such as residronate, pamidronate, clodronate, and tiludronate are being studied by various pharmaceutical companies for their bone-building effects.
- ***Calcitrol***. This powerful version of vitamin D may increase the absorption of calcium and increase levels of calcium in the bloodstream.
- ***Growth factors.*** These substances are produced by osteoblast and other cells. You can think of them as assistants to the osteoblasts. Growth factors help osteoblasts do their work better, and their work is the building of new bone. Doctors hope to learn more about growth factors in order to create a medication that helps the body make more bone.
- ***Sodium fluoride.*** You know that the fluoride in toothpaste makes your teeth stronger, but did you know that it can make your bones stronger as well? Sodium fluoride appears to make bones stronger by attaching itself to the building blocks of calcium that your body uses to create new bone.

- ***Thiazide diuretics***. Also known as water pills, these medications are often used to treat high blood pressure. Doctors are interested in them as a potential treatment for osteoporosis because they have been found to increase calcium levels in the bloodstream.
- ***Parathyroid hormone (PTH).*** This hormone, produced in the body by the parathyroid glands, has a healthy effect on bone in several ways. It increases levels of calcium in the bloodstream, encourages the production of vitamin D, and ultimately spurs the activity of osteoblast cells. Doctors are studying the effects of PTH therapy on osteoporosis, alone and in combination with estrogen.

8

Diet, Exercise, and Alternative Therapies for Osteoporosis

Quick Fact: One cup of milk contains about 300 mg of calcium.

Vanessa, age 32, is a busy mother. She came in to see me for a checkup after the birth of her second child. Her mother had recently been hospitalized following a serious compression fracture of her spine, and Vanessa was concerned that this might happen to her later in life. I explained to Vanessa that she still had three years left to build up her "bone bank account" and that now was an excellent time to begin preventive care. Vanessa did not include much milk or other dairy products in her diet due to lactose intolerance, and since the birth of her second child she had little energy. She also had been taking thyroid hormone for three years, but she had not had her thyroid levels checked in two years. We sat down and together reviewed a positive approach to long-term health. Since increasing Vanessa's intake of dairy products was not a feasible option, she agreed to take 100 mg of calcium with 400 units of vitamin

D each day. Rather than eating salty snacks and drinking caffeinated beverages for energy (both help to dissolve bone), Vanessa agreed to walk with her children for 45 minutes every day. And although she felt tired, a blood test revealed that her thyroid levels were too high, a problem for her bone health. A reduced dose of the thyroid medication made her feel better and strengthened her bones.

Besides the powerful effect it can have on bone building, a program of eating right and regular weight-bearing exercise has plenty of other health benefits. It may reduce your risk of heart disease and cancer and can help relieve stress. Many women are surprised at how good they feel once they start exercising and regret that they did not start sooner. The best approach to fighting osteoporosis at any particular stage of your life depends on your age, how much estrogen is being produced by your ovaries, your medical history, and whether or not you have risk factors. While the aim of this chapter is not to design a diet and exercise program crafted to fit your personal needs, it highlights the aspects of diet and exercise that are important for maintaining healthy bones. Together you and your doctor will craft a specific diet and exercise regimen that is right for you.

As you saw in Chapter 2, the best time to increase the strength of your bones through diet and exercise is before age 30. Your preventive strategy during this time consists of getting adequate dietary calcium (calcium from food or drink) and regular weight-bearing exercise, and eating a nutritious diet. It is during these years that the bone-friendly, construction worker cells called osteoblasts are busy creating new bone by fitting into place building blocks of calcium and other minerals extracted from your bloodstream. Getting enough calcium in your diet and avoiding unhealthy habits such as smoking can make the job of the osteoblasts a lot easier.

As you get older, bone-building activity declines, and the wrecking crew team of cells called osteoclasts starts working overtime to destroy bone. If your bones are strong and resilient, your program of diet and exercise—and possibly calcium or vitamin D supplements—may be enough to stimulate the bone-building osteoblasts and to keep bone weakening at bay by preserving the bone that you already have. In other cases it is not enough. When you have osteoporosis it is critical to keep every ounce of bone that you have and to start on a medication such as Evista (raloxifene) to stem the tide of bone loss. Whatever medication you choose, you will still need to eat a nutritious diet and get the proper amount of exercise. Certain exercises can be very dangerous if you have low bone density because they may increase the risk of a fracture. If you have osteoporosis you should only do those exercises prescribed by your doctor.

Q: How important is calcium?

A: In a word, crucial. The mineral calcium is a key building block used by the osteoblast cells to make bones stronger. Their job is to lay down blocks of calcium in your bones to make them firm. But as you saw in Chapter 1, calcium is a busy and multitalented mineral. Your body uses calcium for other things besides bone building. If you do not get enough calcium in your diet, your body will remove this building block from bone for use in other parts of the body, leaving you with less bone. That is why it is so important to make sure that you get your recommended amount of calcium, no matter what your age. If you get enough calcium, your body will use it to make new bone and have more left over to serve other parts of the body as well. If you are lactose intolerant (have a problem digesting dairy products) it is important that you get calcium from nondairy sources or calcium supplements. Many women with osteoporosis have trouble digesting dairy products, and this may explain why they had trouble getting enough dietary calcium. See Chapter 2 for a chart showing how much calcium you need.

Q: I am a woman in my early thirties and am very conscientious about getting enough calcium in my diet. But how do I know if I am getting enough vitamin D?

A: That is a good question. As you saw in Chapter 1, calcium and vitamin D go hand in hand. They are the dynamic duo that fights bone loss. Vitamin D actually helps the body to use more of the calcium that you get from food or drink. Before menopause, most women do not have to worry about getting enough vitamin D. The body manufactures vitamin D in response to direct sunlight, so getting 15 minutes or so of sunshine every day usually stimulates the production of necessary amounts. Women below age 40 who are physically active and outdoors much of the time probably do not need any vitamin D supplementation, but women who are mostly indoors or live in the north would probably benefit from some supplementation. You are probably getting the daily recommended 400 international units (IU) of vitamin D through your diet. Taking a multivitamin that contains vitamin D is another way of making sure that you are getting enough, though most women your age do not need vitamin D supplements—in fact, too much vitamin D can actually cause bone loss. In addition to calcium and vitamin D, there are other vitamins and minerals that you need for maintaining healthy bones. These include vitamin K, vitamin B_{12}, vitamin C, vitamin A, magnesium,

Good Sources of Dietary Calcium

Food	Amount	Approximate calcium content (mg)
Dairy		
Whole milk	1 cup	290
2% milk	1 cup	300
1% milk	1 cup	300
Skim milk	1 cup	302
Buttermilk	1 cup	285
Low-fat yogurt	1 cup	415
Cheddar cheese	1 oz	205
Monterey Jack cheese	1 oz	212
Mozzarella cheese, skim	1 oz	207
Muenster cheese	1 oz	203
Seafood		
Oysters	1 cup	225
Mackerel, canned	3 oz	205
Sardines, with bones	3 oz	370
Salmon, with bones	3 oz	167
Vegetables		
Broccoli, cooked	1 cup	136
Turnip greens, cooked	1 cup	250
Collard greens, cooked	1 cup	357
Dandelion greens, cooked	1 cup	280
Mustard greens, cooked	1 cup	276
Kale	1 cup	180

continued

Food	Amount	Approximate calcium content (mg)
Fruits, nuts, and beans		
Almonds	¼ cup	94
Brazil nuts	¼ cup	62
Hazelnuts	¼ cup	55
Tofu	4 oz	108
Beans, dried, cooked	1 cup	90

boron, and zinc. You can get these vitamins and minerals by eating a balanced, nutritious diet such as that outlined in the Food Guide Pyramid (see page 140) or by taking a multivitamin containing the recommended daily allowance (RDA) of these nutrients.

Q: Why are calcium and vitamin D supplements important as women age?

A: As your body loses estrogen due to menopause, it becomes less efficient at absorbing dietary calcium and turning it into the building blocks of bone. This is a problem because most women do not get enough calcium in their diets in the first place. The body also tends to manufacture less vitamin D as estrogen levels go down, so less calcium is available for the body's use. New medical studies suggest that vitamin D deficiency may play a greater role in the development of osteoporosis than was previously thought. A 1998 study in the *New England Journal of Medicine* suggests that many Americans lack sufficient amounts of vitamin D in the blood needed to adequately protect against bone loss. In another study of 160 people between the ages of 49 and 83 who visited hospital clinics of the Boston University

Good Sources of Vitamin D

- Chicken liver
- Egg yolks
- Fish liver oils
- Fortified milk
- Herring
- Salmon
- Sardines
- Swiss cheese

Medical Center, 40% were deficient in vitamin D. The women in these studies who had low levels of vitamin D probably did not get enough of it through diet or supplements or did not get out in the sun enough—and direct sunlight is necessary in order to stimulate the body's production of the vitamin. Increased use of sunblock during the summer has also contributed to decreased sun exposure and may help to explain why some women have vitamin D deficiency.

Q: Is it true that eating meat can weaken bones?

A: A healthy diet often means eating certain foods in moderation. That is the case with meat. Meat is a great source of protein—though not the only source, as any vegetarian will tell you—and protein is very important to your health. It helps to grow and repair tissue in the body and also forms the basis for new bone. But while eating meat is crucial to the formation of new bone, eating too much meat can actually weaken bone. The problem with meat is that it is acidic. When you have too much meat in your diet, your body tries to balance the high level of acidity by removing minerals like calcium from your bloodstream. If there is not enough calcium in your blood, your body automatically removes calcium building blocks from your bones and sends them back into your bloodstream, leaving you with less bone. Most women do not get enough calcium in their diets in the first place, so eating too much meat can make the situation even worse. This does not mean that you have to stop eating meat. Just try to limit your consumption of meat to 4 to 9 ounces of cooked lean meat a day. If you get most of your protein from nonmeat sources, this is not a problem that you have to worry about.

Q: My doctor told me years ago to avoid salt because it may lead to high blood pressure. Is it true that too much salt can also make my bones weaker?

A: Yes, so you now have two good reasons to cut back on sodium, commonly referred to as salt. This mineral is necessary to help keep body fluids in proper balance. But most people simply get too much of it. It has been known for some time that too much sodium can increase your risk for high blood pressure. Research now suggests that sodium may also contribute to bone loss by increasing loss of calcium in the urine. Your goal should be to keep the amount of sodium you consume below 2,400 mg a day (this is roughly the amount of sodium in a teaspoon of table salt). As you probably know, this is easier said than done because sodium is found in high amounts in the foods that many Americans love to eat.

Most women get sodium from two sources—the salt shaker and from food prepared with high amounts of sodium. In order to cut down on sodium, do not reach so often for the table salt at meals; use it sparingly. You will find that the less you use salt, the less you will crave it. You should also avoid foods that are high in sodium such as most snack foods (sorry, potato chip lovers); fast food; canned vegetables or other goods; sandwich meats such as bologna, salami, or corned beef; and Chinese and other take-out foods that contain monosodium glutamate (MSG)—most restaurants will prepare your food without MSG if you ask them to. Try eating fresh vegetables instead of canned, using sandwich meats that are low in sodium (often advertised on the label), and preparing more food at home instead of relying on take-out or burgers and fries.

Q: I read somewhere that alcohol may help to prevent heart disease. Is it good for the bones as well?

A: That sounds like wishful thinking, but the answer is no. Although it does appear that drinking alcohol in moderation can help prevent heart disease to some degree, we know with more certainty that even a little alcohol in your diet can do a double whammy on your bones by interfering with the way your body uses calcium and vitamin D—the dynamic duo that fights bone loss. Drinking too much alcohol also goes hand in hand with other unhealthy habits; if you are drinking heavily you are probably not getting enough exercise or eating properly, either. It is also thought that the protein deficiency associated with alcoholism can contribute to the development of osteoporosis. Heavy drinking, even when not linked to protein deficiency, may slow down the work of the bone-building osteoblasts and have a negative effect on the bone-remodeling process. The best advice is to stop drinking alcohol or at the very least limit yourself to two drinks a day—less if possible. See Chapter 9 for information on other ways to help prevent heart disease.

Q: What does coffee have to do with osteoporosis?

A: This may not be good news for those women who depend on several cups of coffee to get through the day. Caffeine may give you an extra burst of energy but it is definitely not bone friendly. In fact, it reduces the amount of calcium available for building new bone. Give up coffee or tea altogether or switch to a decaffeinated brand. Otherwise, be sure to drink less than three cups of coffee or seven cups of tea a day. Too many women think that taking their coffee or tea with milk may help to compensate for the calcium that they are losing due to caffeine. That is a poor way to supplement.

Q: I remember a time when the four food groups were all you needed to know about eating right. I am not sure I know what a healthy diet is these days. Can you help?

A: Fortunately, doctors know more about eating right today than they ever did, and it is not as complicated as you may think. While the purpose of this chapter is not to offer a specific diet regimen, we can look at the U.S. Department of Agriculture's (USDA) relatively simple recommendations for healthy eating summarized in the Food Guide Pyramid. You can think of it as a new and improved version of the famous four food groups. The general guidelines for a healthy diet according to the Food Guide Pyramid are described below. As you can see, the basic idea is to eat more grains, fruits, and vegetables and to go easy on the meat, dairy products, and fats. But keep in mind that dairy products are typically good sources of calcium. The USDA recommends that you eat at least the lowest numbers of servings from each of the groups listed below in order to get proper amounts of vitamins, minerals, carbohydrates, and protein.

- ***Bread, cereal, rice, and pasta (6 to 11 servings a day).*** A serving is one slice of bread, 1 ounce of cereal, or ½ cup of cooked cereal, rice, or pasta.
- ***Vegetables (3 to 5 servings a day).*** A serving is 1 cup of raw, leafy vegetables; ½ cup of other vegetables, cooked or chopped raw; or ¾ cup of vegetable juice.
- ***Fruit (2 to 4 servings a day).*** A serving is one medium apple, banana, or orange; ½ cup of chopped, cooked, or canned fruit; or ¾ cup of fruit juice.
- ***Meat, poultry, fish, dried beans, eggs, and nuts (2 to 3 servings a day).*** A serving is 2 to 3 ounces of cooked lean meat, poultry, or fish; ½ cup of cooked dried beans, one egg, or 2 tablespoons of peanut butter count as 1 ounce of lean meat.
- ***Milk, yogurt, and cheese (2 to 3 servings a day).*** A serving is 1 cup of milk or yogurt, 1½ ounces of natural cheese, or 2 ounces of processed cheese.
- ***Fats, oils, and sweets.*** Use sparingly.

Q: What are the benefits of exercise?

A: Exercise—specifically the weight-bearing variety—can increase bone density during the peak bone-building years and help to preserve bone as you grow older. That makes it very important. In fact, weight-bearing exercise is better at increasing bone density than any other kind of fitness activity. Though many women lift weights these days, weight-bearing exercises do not necessarily

The USDA's Food Guide Pyramid: A guide to daily food choices

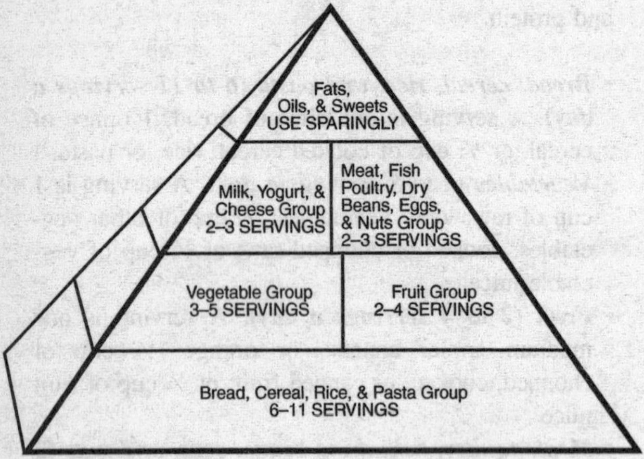

Source: U.S. Department of Agriculture/U.S. Department of Health and Human Services

involve pumping iron in a sweaty gym. Walking, jogging, hiking, aerobic routines, stair climbing, jumping rope, and bicycling or using a stationary bike also strengthen bones. Cross-country skiing, tennis, basketball, and racquetball all have bone-building benefits as well. The trick is to experiment with different kinds of exercise until you find those that you enjoy and that you can do on a regular basis. Women who exercise with a partner often find it easier to stick to their workout. Besides its effects on bone, exercise can strengthen your muscles, improve your coordination and balance, and make you more flexible. These benefits make you less likely to fall or more able to prevent a fall from becoming a serious injury. Most doctors recommend that you exercise three days a week for 30 to 60 minutes a day.

Q: Is it safe to exercise if I already have osteoporosis?

A: Yes, although great care must be taken when exercising with very low bone density. Only your doctor can adequately say what level of exercise is right for you. Your doctor knows your medical history and what medications you may be taking, and these are important factors in shaping a workout program. You cannot necessarily follow the same exercise regimen that you and your doctor devised when trying to *prevent* osteoporosis, because doing this may actually cause an injury. It is especially important to consult your doctor if you have suffered any sort of fracture—particularly a hip fracture or a recent vertebral fracture. But even after a fracture, your doctor will encourage you to begin exercising as soon as possible at a level that is safe for you. Exercising with osteoporosis usually involves a walking program, strength training exercises (for the hips, back, thighs, and arms), and exercises to improve balance and coordination. Your doctor may also recommend spine-extension exercises, in which the spine is arched back, that build muscles in the back and strengthen the spine itself.

In general, certain exercises are considered unsafe for women with low bone density. Any type of exercise that involves bending or twisting—this is termed *flexion exercise* by doctors—is off limits when you have osteoporosis (or have already had a osteoporosis-related fracture) because it can cause compression fractures in the spine. Sports like golf, tennis, bowling, and racquetball fall into this category. Even sit-ups and toe touches are risky activities. It is also important not to perform any activity that puts stress on the spine itself, such as jumping, high-impact aerobics, or jogging. Exercises that require moving the legs sideways, particularly against resistance, can put dangerous stress on the hip.

Q: I have heard that soy foods may actually help to prevent osteoporosis. Is that true?

A: As of now, we simply do not know. As you saw in Chapter 6, there is some evidence suggesting that soy foods may help to alleviate some of the symptoms of menopause. Soy foods may have this effect because they contain phytoestrogens. Phytoestrogens are estrogen-like substances found naturally in certain plants. These substances are found in soy products (such as soy milk, tofu, roasted soy nuts, soy flour, and tempeh), flax seeds, and some herbs. It is unclear whether or not these weak estrogens can have an effect on slowing bone loss. In one study, six months of a high-soy diet appeared to increase bone density. Some doctors even think that phytoestrogens may have the ability to selectively mimic the effects of estrogen. As you saw in Chapter 4, Evista increases bone density and may even offer protection against breast cancer because of its ability to act like estrogen in some parts of the body while blocking the effects of estrogen in others. Could phytoestrogens be nature's equivalent of Evista and other selective estrogen receptor modulators (SERMs)? No one knows for sure. Several studies suggest that soy foods may in fact have a protective effect against breast cancer and may also lower cholesterol levels. Soy foods are also high in calcium, which is essential for building strong bones. While the data is intriguing, it is simply too early to speculate as to whether soy foods or plants containing phytoestrogens can help fight osteoporosis or heart disease or make breast cancer less likely. We also do not know enough about the risks of taking large amounts of phytoestrogens.

9

The Future of Evista and SERMs: Treating Heart Disease and Breast Cancer

Quick Fact: Heart disease is the number one killer of American women.

Joanne, age 48, had three older sisters who all developed breast cancer in their early fifties. Her menstrual cycles were becoming irregular, and she was noticing some irritability and hot flashes just before her periods. Joanne was well informed at our visit and was concerned about her health after menopause. She was very concerned about using hormone replacement therapy (HRT) because of her family history of breast cancer, but she felt that something other than proper diet and regular exercise would be necessary to combat osteoporosis and heart disease as she got older. I agreed that because of the risks of long-term HRT and her fears about breast cancer, we would need to consider choices other than estrogen therapy. I ordered a bone density test that was normal and a serum cholesterol test that was a healthy 168. I explained to Joanne that at the moment no treatment was needed. After menopause, Evista might be a good choice because studies indicate that it may provide protection against breast cancer while preventing other health risks associated with aging. However, given her excellent health, there was no hurry to begin treatment, and future selective estrogen receptor modulators (SERMs) might have even greater protective effects against bone weakening and breast cancer. We agreed to maximize diet and exercise in the meantime and review new research and medication options at each annual visit.

Imagine a medication that helps to fight osteoporosis and heart disease, eases hot flashes and other troublesome menopausal symptoms, and can be used to prevent breast cancer in the bargain—and it accomplishes all this with few side effects. Sound too good to be true? Perhaps. But as fantastic as it sounds, this is the future that some doctors are predicting for selective estrogen receptor modulators (SERMs). Evista (raloxifene) and other SERMs may very well change the way that doctors and the American public look at the idea of hormonal therapy. The mainstay of hormonal therapy for women during and after menopause has long been estrogen replacement therapy (ERT)—in which a form of estrogen made in a laboratory is used to replace the estrogen lost during menopause—or hormone replacement therapy (HRT)—in which estrogen is given along with progesterone in order to reduce the risk of cancer of the uterus. Despite the benefits of estrogen therapy, many women choose not to use it for fears that it may cause breast or uterine cancer or unwanted side effects.

Evista and SERMs have changed this relatively simple picture of what hormonal therapy can be. As you saw in

Chapter 4, Evista and other SERMs are like chemical copycats. They act like estrogen in some parts of the body where estrogen has a healthy effect and block estrogen's effects in other parts where the presence of estrogen may be harmful. SERMs are often referred to as "designer estrogens" or "second-generation estrogens" because many doctors believe that they are a technological advance over standard hormonal therapy. Estrogen therapy is a way of restoring lost estrogen. It does not make decisions about when to act like estrogen and when not to. By selectively imitating estrogen, SERMs of the future may be able to deliver all the benefits of estrogen while minimizing the risks or side effects.

What is the future of SERMs? No one knows for certain. But in some cases that future may be sooner than you think. SERMs that are already available to the public, such as Evista and tamoxifen (Nolvadex), are already showing signs that they may be used in the near future in ways other than those for which they are approved by the Food and Drug Administration (FDA). Tamoxifen has recently been approved by the FDA for reducing the risk of breast cancer and both medications are being studied for their healthy effects on the heart. Evista may be just the beginning of this fascinating search for a "miracle" menopause medication. Doctors are hard at work in the laboratories of major pharmaceutical companies where they are trying to design custom-made SERMs for use in the relatively near future. As of late 1998, at least seven other SERMs are being studied. These new SERMs, doctors hope, will be even more successful at copying the full range of estrogen's healthy effects, such as its ability to ease menopausal symptoms and protect women from Alzheimer's disease. See Chapter 4 for more information on how SERMs work.

Q: I thought that heart disease was a man's problem. Is this something that I need to worry about after menopause?

A: Heart disease is definitely not just a man's problem, especially for women who have completed menopause. You may be surprised to learn that heart disease is the number one killer of American women. In fact, six to ten years after menopause, women have just about as many heart attacks as do men—this is not exactly the sort of equality most women are looking for. Cardiovascular disease kills about 500,000 women a year, and about half of those deaths are due to heart attacks. By way of comparison, breast cancer claims the lives of about 43,000 women a year. The consequences of heart attacks are also more serious in women. About 44% of women who have heart attacks die within a year compared to 27% of men. The future health outlook for women who do survive heart attacks is not encouraging either. According to the Framingham Heart Study, within six years after a heart attack, 31% of women will have another heart attack, 34% will develop angina, 18% will have a stroke, 20% will be disabled by heart failure (heart failure is discussed later in the chapter), and 6% will experience sudden death. These figures are not intended to frighten you. But they should impress you with the fact that heart disease is an important health concern that every postmenopausal women must take seriously.

Q: What exactly is heart disease?

A: Usually when we talk about heart disease we are really talking about coronary heart disease (CHD), the type of heart disease associated with heart attack. In CHD, an artery that supplies the heart with blood becomes thickened and hardened due to a buildup of cholesterol and other substances (including calcium) in the lining of the artery. This buildup is called plaque (not to be confused with the sort of plaque that accumulates on your teeth). This thickening and hardening of the arteries is referred to by doctors as atherosclerosis—from the Greek *athero* (''gruel'' or ''paste'') and *sclerosis* (''hardening''). This plaque may partially or totally block the blood's flow through an artery. A dangerous blood clot—called a *thrombus* by doctors—may also form on the surface of the plaque. Either of these situations can have very serious consequences for your heart. When the heart is deprived of adequate oxygen due to lack of blood supply, it cannot pump effectively. This may lead in some cases to the chronic chest pain and shortness of breath associated with angina. In more serious cases, the result is a heart attack, in which areas of the heart actually die because they are starved for oxygen.

Q: What is congestive heart failure?

A: Congestive heart failure (CHF)—also known simply as heart failure—is another dangerous kind of heart disease. CHF occurs when the heart cannot pump enough blood to meet the needs of the body's other organs. This can result from CHD, high blood pressure, heart valve disease, or from other causes. In CHF, the heart does not work as well as it should and the flow of blood being pumped out of the heart slows down. Women with CHF often cannot exert themselves because they become short of breath and tired. They usually have swelling—called edema by doctors—in the legs and ankles and sometimes in other parts of the body as well. Fluid may also collect in the lungs and interfere with normal breathing.

Top Five Causes of Death in American Women

1. Heart disease
2. Cancer
3. Cerebrovascular diseases
4. Chronic obstructive pulmonary diseases and allied conditions
5. Pneumonia and influenza

Source: R. N. Anderson, K. D. Kochanek, and S. L. Murphy. Report of Final Mortality Statistics, 1995. *Monthly Vital Statistics Report*; vol 45; no. 11; supp 2.

CHF may not be as dramatic as a heart attack but it is disabling and life-threatening. After CHF is diagnosed, only about 15% of women survive longer than 8 to 12 years. Heart transplants are the only option for survival in some cases.

Q: Can Evista really help to prevent heart disease?

A: While Evista has not been approved by the FDA for treating heart disease, Evista has shown some beneficial effects on the heart. Studies suggest that Evista may be able to lower total blood cholesterol levels and levels of low density lipoprotein (LDL) cholesterol—the so-called ''bad'' cholesterol—in postmenopausal women. This means that Evista may be effective in preventing heart disease. In the 24-month osteoporosis prevention trials discussed in Chapter 5, doctors also looked at the effect that Evista had on cholesterol levels. Compared to a placebo (sugar pill), Evista lowered total blood cholesterol by about 5% and LDL cholesterol by about 8%. Evista did not have any effect on levels of high density lipoprotein (HDL) cholesterol—the so-called "good" cholesterol. So does taking Evista help to prevent heart attacks? Unfortunately, doctors do not know the answer to that question, but many doctors think that it will. As of early 1999, studies were ongoing to determine whether Evista could reduce the number of heart attacks in postmenopausal women. It is likely that Evista will be approved by the FDA for preventing heart disease in the next several years.

Q: How does Evista help to protect against heart disease?

A: A better question might be, "How does estrogen help to fight heart disease?" Doctors think that Evista acts like estrogen in the cardiovascular system, which explains why it may have a healthy effect. Doctors assume that the loss of estrogen during menopause is one major reason why postmenopausal women are at increased risk of heart attack. They are less sure about how estrogen works its magic in the cardiovascular system. But doctors do have some theories. We know that there are estrogen receptors in the arteries, where plaque tends to build up. As you saw in Chapter 1, estrogen binds to receptors in order to deliver messages that have an effect on the tissue in that area. This suggests that estrogen "locks in" to these receptors and delivers messages that ultimately help to maintain healthy cardiovascular tissue. For example, estrogen may enhance the effectiveness of the healthier fats in the bloodstream or block the narrowing effect of certain chemicals. It may even help to prevent the buildup of plaque on artery walls or increase the flow of blood, which helps to wash away fatty buildup. By acting like estrogen, Evista appears to have a healthy effect on the heart.

Q: What is cholesterol?

A: Cholesterol is a soft, fatty substance. It is one of the fats in the bloodstream—called *lipids* by doctors—and is found in all your body's cells. Cholesterol is necessary to maintain good health. It is used to make cell membranes and sex hormones. Cholesterol comes from two sources. It is produced by your body (mostly in the liver) and is also found in foods that come from animals, such as meats, poultry, fish, seafood, and dairy products. Foods from plants do not contain cholesterol. The problem with cholesterol is that most women simply have too much of it, and that can be bad for your heart. When you get too much cholesterol, it can lead to the formation of plaque. This can cause thickening and hardening of the arteries, which reduces the flow of blood to the heart. A high cholesterol level is a major risk factor for CHD. The American Heart Association (AHA) recommends that you limit your average daily intake of dietary cholesterol (the cholesterol that you get from food or drink) to 300 mg. By reducing your dietary cholesterol, you can lessen your risk of heart disease.

Total blood cholesterol is the most common measurement of blood cholesterol. It is the number you usually receive as test results from your doctor. When you hear someone say, "My doctor told me I need to get my cholesterol down below 200," that person is referring to a total blood cholesterol measurement. Knowing your total blood cholesterol level is an important first step in determining your risk for heart disease. And a woman's blood cholesterol tends to increase with age, according to the AHA. For example, before age 45, total blood cholesterol in women ranges from 185 to 207 mg/dL, while between the ages of 45 and 64 it rises to somewhere between 217 to 237 mg/dL. The higher your total blood cholesterol level, the higher your heart disease risk. For all adults, a desirable total blood cholesterol level is less than 200 mg/dL. A level of 240 mg/dL or above is considered high blood cholesterol. But even levels in the "borderline high" category (200 to 239 mg/dL) boost the risk of heart disease.

Q: What is the difference between LDL and HDL cholesterol?

A: In simple terms, lipoproteins are proteins that transport fats like cholesterol. Cholesterol does not dissolve in your blood. It must be transported by other substances. These substances are the lipoproteins. You can think of lipoproteins as freight trains riding the rails of your bloodstream. The main cargo that they are hauling is cholesterol. LDL cholesterol is the main carrier of cholesterol in the blood. It tends to unload its cargo of cholesterol right onto the walls of your arteries, where it may build up and form plaques unless it is removed by HDL cholesterol. That explains why LDL cholesterol is called the "bad" cholesterol. A high level of LDL cholesterol in the blood means you may be at a high risk for a heart attack. An LDL level below 130 mg/dL is desirable, while levels of 130 to 159 mg/dL are borderline-high. LDL levels of 160 mg/dL or above mean you have a high risk of developing CHD. Although an LDL cholesterol measurement is not necessary for your first cholesterol test, your doctor may recommend that you have your LDL cholesterol level

Risk Factors for CHD

Risk factors that you can change	Risk factors that you cannot change
High blood pressure	Gender
High blood cholesterol	Heredity
Smoking	Age
Obesity	
Physical inactivity	
Diabetes	
Stress	

checked after reviewing your initial test results and your medical history. HDL cholesterol is known as the "good" cholesterol. It transports less fat than does LDL cholesterol but moves in an opposite and healthier direction. HDL cholesterol tends to carry its cholesterol cargo away from the arteries and back to the liver, where it is passed from the body or used to make other substances. By removing excess cholesterol from plaque, HDL cholesterol may slow its growth. Having a high level of HDL cholesterol means that you may have a lower risk of a heart attack. If your HDL level is less than 35 mg/dL, your risk of heart disease goes up.

Q: Is it true that some fats are good for my health and others are bad?

A: It is true that certain fats are better for you than others, but it is also important to realize that too much of any kind of fat is unhealthy. The trick is knowing which is which. There are two main kinds of fat. Both are found in almost all foods in varying amounts. The fat that you should avoid is called *saturated fat*. Saturated fat can raise your blood cholesterol level, so cutting back on foods that contain this type of fat is a great way to help lower your risk of heart disease. Unfortunately, saturated fat is found in high amounts in many of our favorite foods. Some of these foods come from animals and others are made from plants. Foods that come from animals and contain large amounts of saturated fat include beef, pork, veal, poultry, butter, cream, whole milk, and cheese and other dairy products made from whole milk. These foods also contain dietary cholesterol, so they do a double whammy on your heart. Foods from plants that contain high amounts of saturated fat include coconut oil, palm kernel oil, and palm oil—also known as tropical oils (do not be fooled by the pleasant-sounding name)—and cocoa butter. Unfortunately, these oils are often cheaper than the alternatives and therefore are used by many companies that make processed foods and snack foods such as potato chips.

But all fats are not created equal. On the other end of the scale there are fats that may actually have a healthy effect on your heart. These fats are called *unsaturated fats*. There are two kinds of unsaturated fat—polyunsaturated and monounsaturated. Polyunsaturated fat is found in many cooking oils and in margarine. Polyunsaturated fat is found in safflower, sunflower, and sesame seeds, soybeans and corn, certain nuts, and in the oils made from these. Polyunsaturated fat appears to help the body get rid of newly deposited cholesterol, so this type of fat may help to lower your blood cholesterol and reduce plaque. Monounsaturated fat is found in olive, canola, and peanut oils and in avocados. This type of fat may also help to reduce your blood cholesterol level as long as your diet is very low in saturated fat. But just because unsaturated fats may have a healthy effect on your heart does not mean that you can eat as much of them as you want. Like every part of your diet, moderation is the key. It is important to limit the amount of total fat that you eat each day, regardless of what type of fat it is. So how much is too much? That depends on how many calories you consume each day. Based on an 1,800-calorie-a-day diet (which is what the average woman gets), you should consume no more than 60 g of fat a day. Of those 60 g, you should consume no more than 18 g of saturated fat a day. Read food labels to find out how much fat is contained in the foods you eat.

Q: What can I do to help prevent heart disease?

A: In addition to keeping your bones healthy, a proper diet (one that is low in cholesterol and in saturated fat) and regular exercise can help to prevent heart disease—as can eliminating unhealthy habits. First of all, if you smoke, stop! The risk of heart attack in women who smoke is more than twice that of nonsmokers, and smokers who have heart attacks are more likely to die from them. Even secondhand smoke increases your risk. In women who are overweight, losing some of that weight may help to reduce your risk of heart disease by lowering LDL cholesterol and boosting HDL cholesterol. Aerobic-type exercises that get the heart pumping are also important because they help to condition the heart and may also increase HDL cholesterol in some women. These exercises, which should be done on a regular basis, include brisk walking, jogging, bicycling, jumping rope, aerobic dance, and swimming. Even mild-intensity

Tips for Planning Meals That are Healthy for Your Heart

- Choose fish, poultry, and lean cuts of meat, and remove the fat and skin before eating.
- Broil, bake, roast, and poach foods instead of frying them.
- Cut down on high-fat processed meats, including sausage, bacon, and such cold cuts as salami and bologna. (These foods often contain high amounts of sodium, which as you saw in Chapter 8 is also bad for your bones.)
- Limit organ meats, such as liver, kidney, and brain.
- Use low- or nonfat milk and cheeses, and low- or nonfat yogurt.
- Instead of butter, use liquid or soft margarine or vegetable oils high in unsaturated fats. Use all fats and oils sparingly.
- Eat egg yolks only in moderation. Egg whites contain no fat or cholesterol and can be eaten often.
- Eat plenty of fruits and vegetables, as well as cereals, breads, rice, and pasta made from enriched or whole grains.
- Get in the habit of reading food labels. Many packaged and processed foods are high in saturated fat. Look for the ''Nutrition Facts'' chart on the label and choose products that are lowest in fat and saturated fat. Also read products for cholesterol content.

Source: Adapted from the National Heart, Lung, and Blood Institute (NHLBI).

activities, if done daily, can help reduce your risk of heart disease. Taking an evening stroll, gardening, doing yard work and housework, and dancing all may have benefits for your cardiovascular system. You may not even think of some of these activities as exercise in the classic sense of the word, yet they can help you to keep your heart healthy. Exercise can also help to control diabetes and combat obesity and high blood pressure—all three of these are also risk factors for heart disease.

Q: Is it true that alcohol can help to prevent heart disease?
A: It appears to be true. In some studies, moderate use of alcohol is linked with higher HDL levels. The incidence of heart disease for women who drink one glass of alcohol a day is lower than in nondrinkers. But the benefit is not great enough to recommend drinking alcohol if you do not drink already. According to a large study published in 1997 by the American Cancer Society (ACS), having one drink a day raises a woman's risk of dying of breast cancer by 11%. Alcohol also is associated with a host of other health problems such as osteoporosis, alcoholism, obesity, high blood pressure, stroke, and suicide. It is best to talk to your doctor about whether or not it is a good idea to drink alcohol in moderation if at all. Your doctor knows your medical history and can help you determine whether it is in your best interest, depending on the state of your health, any existing medical conditions (such as osteoporosis), and your specific health concerns.

Q: What is breast cancer?
A: Cancer is the uncontrolled growth of abnormal cells, often forming a tumor, that invade and destroy healthy

Calorie-Burning Activities That May Help You to Maintain a Healthy Weight

Activity	Calories Burned per Hour*
Light Activity	
• Cleaning the house	240
• Playing golf	
Moderate Activity	
• Brisk walking (3.5 mph)	370
• Gardening	
• Bicycling (5.5 mph)	
Strenuous Activity	
• Jogging (9 min. per mile)	580
• Swimming	
Very Strenuous Activity	
• Running (7 min. per mile)	740
• Skiing	

*For a healthy, 140-lb. woman.

Source: *Dietary Guidelines for Americans*, U.S. Department of Agriculture (USDA), 1990.

tissue. Breast cancer is a malignant tumor that develops in breast tissue. Sometimes cancerous cells detach from the tumor and travel through the bloodstream to other areas of the body where they continue to do damage—doctors call this a metastasis. Breast cancer occurs mostly in women and only rarely in men. It is the leading cause of cancer death among women between the ages of 40 and 55 and is the second leading cause of cancer death among all women (lung cancer being the first). Several factors can increase your risk of this type of cancer. First of all, breast cancer risk increases with age. Almost 7% of women over age 60 develop breast cancer. The risk is also higher in women who have had breast cancer in the past or who have a family history of breast cancer. The timing of important moments in your reproductive life also plays a role. Women who began having menstrual periods at an early age or who experienced menopause late in life are more likely to develop breast cancer, as is a woman who has never had children or had her first child at a late age. Recent use of birth control pills or estrogen therapy can also increase your risk. Other risk factors still being studied include exposure to pesticides and other chemicals, alcohol use, weight gain, a high-fat diet, and a sedentary lifestyle.

Q: What are the symptoms of breast cancer?

A: Breast cancer often shows up as an abnormality on a mammogram before you or your doctor can feel it. When breast cancer progresses to the point where symptoms do exist, these may include a breast lump, swelling or tenderness, and nipple pain. Contrary to what some women believe, having breast pain is not usually a sign of cancer. In fact, the opposite is often true. Breast pain usually means that you have a benign (noncancerous) condition. It rarely is an early symptom of breast cancer. The ACS recommends that women over age 39 have mammograms every year and that women over age 19 perform breast self-examinations every month in order to help detect breast cancer. The thinking is that by doing the self-examination regularly, you will get to know how your breasts normally feel. This way, you can more readily find anything out of the ordinary. You should not be alarmed if you notice a change in your breasts (though you should tell your doctor about it). Just because you find an irregularity does not mean that you have breast cancer.

Q: Can Evista really prevent breast cancer?

A: The jury is still out, but Evista certainly has exciting potential as a possible chemopreventive agent. This is the term that doctors use for any medication or other substance that has the ability to prevent cancer from developing. What evidence do we have that Evista may someday be used as a preventive medication for breast cancer? In a number of short-term studies, women who took Evista did not develop breast cancer as often as women who took a placebo. Study results reported in early 1998 suggest that Evista may protect postmenopausal women from developing breast cancer by as much as 50%. In an earlier 30-month study, there was a 62% decrease in the expected incidence of breast cancer among those who took Evista, which also suggests that it might provide protection for the breast. Unlike tamoxifen, Evista does *not* appear to act like an estrogen in the uterus and has not been linked to an increase in endometrial cancer.

One recent study, the Multiple Outcomes of Evista Evaluation (MORE) trial, even suggests that Evista may

How to Do a Breast Self-Examination

By regularly examining your own breasts, you are likely to notice any changes that occur. The best time for breast self-examination is about a week after your period ends, when your breasts are not tender or swollen. If you are not having regular periods, do a breast self-examination on the same day every month.

1. Lie down with a pillow under your right shoulder and place your right arm behind your head.
2. Use the finger pads of the three middle fingers on your left hand to feel for lumps in the right breast.
3. Press firmly enough to know how your breast feels. A firm ridge in the lower curve of each breast is normal. If you are not sure how hard to press, ask your doctor.
4. Move around the breast in a circular, up-and-down line, or wedge pattern. Be sure to do it the same way every time. Check the entire breast area and remember how your breast feels from month to month.
5. Repeat the exam on your left breast, using the finger pads of the right hand. (Move the pillow under your left shoulder.)
6. If you find any changes, see your doctor right away.
7. Repeat the examination of both breasts while standing, with one arm behind your head. The upright position makes it easier to check the upper and outer part of the breasts (toward your armpit).

This is where about half of breast cancers are found. You may want to do the standing part of the exam while you are in the shower. Some breast changes can be felt more easily when your skin is wet and soapy.

8. For added safety, you can check your breasts for any dimpling of the skin, changes in the nipple, redness, or swelling while standing in front of a mirror right after your exam each month.

Source: Reprinted by the permission of American Cancer Society, Inc.

help to *prevent* cancer of the uterus while reducing the risk of breast cancer. The MORE trial involved almost 8,000 postmenopausal women with osteoporosis who were given Evista (60 or 120 mg) or a placebo. Three years of Evista reduced the risk of breast cancer by about 70% in this study and appeared to reduce the risk of endometrial cancer as well—regardless of whether women took 60 mg or 120 mg dosages of the medication. While the above findings may inspire women with hope, some doctors are taking a conservative view about Evista's possible preventive effects on the breast. This is primarily due to the fact that Evista has not been studied long enough to accurately gauge whether or not it prevents breast cancer. At this point is looks promising but further research needs to be done over a period of years.

Q: Is tamoxifen a SERM, too?

A: Yes. Tamoxifen is the most widely used therapy for the treatment of breast cancer. Doctors have been prescribing it for 20 years and it is used to treat women with all stages of the disease. In late 1998 tamoxifen was approved by the FDA for reducing the risk of breast cancer in women who are likely to develop the disease due to family history or other reasons—the first medication ever to make such a claim. Tamoxifen is thought to block the effect of estrogen in breast tissue, where estrogen seems to promote the growth of cancerous cells. Tamoxifen also is being studied to determine whether it is useful in the treatment of other types of cancer, such as cancer of the uterus, melanoma, and leukemia. Tamoxifen acts like estrogen in other parts of the body as well, making it something of a double-edged sword. It appears to have a healthy effect on the heart and bones by lowering blood cholesterol levels and slowing bone loss. Unfortunately, tamoxifen also appears to act like estrogen in the uterus, where the presence of estrogen can increase the risk of cancer. Several studies suggest that women taking tamoxifen as a treatment for breast cancer face a risk of uterine cancer about two to three times higher than the risk for women who do not take it.

Q: What is the Breast Cancer Prevention Trial?

A: An important study for women concerned about breast cancer. The National Surgical Adjuvant Breast and Bowel Project (NSABP) Breast Cancer Prevention Trial involved over 13,000 women age 35 or over at high risk for breast cancer. These women took tamoxifen or a placebo for 4 or 5 years. Age is such an important risk factor for breast cancer that women age 60 or over were allowed to participate in the trial based on their age alone. Younger women were eligible if they had certain combinations of risk factors. The trial was stopped 14 months early (in early 1998) to give women in the placebo group a chance to switch to tamoxifen. Why stop the trial? After about 5 years of study tamoxifen was found to reduce the risk of breast cancer by almost 50%. The study results were published in the *Journal of the National Cancer Institute* in 1998. Women in the tamoxifen group had fewer bone fractures of the hip, wrist, and spine that women in the placebo group, but tamoxifen did not reduce heart attack risk. It *did* increase the risk of cancer of the uterus and of potentially dangerous blood clots. The decision of the FDA to approve tamoxifen as a risk reducer was based largely on the results of this study.

Q: Is it true that there is a new breast cancer prevention trial underway that compares tamoxifen to Evista?

A: Yes. The NSABP Study of Tamoxifen and Raloxifene (STAR), a large-scale clinical trial in which two SERMs will go head-to-head as risk reducers, is scheduled to open at over 400 sites across the United States and Canada in 1999. This seven-year study will involve 22,000 healthy, postmenopausal women at increased risk for developing breast cancer. Women who qualify for participation in STAR must be age 35 or over and must be considered at high risk for the disease based on a variety of factors. These include age, the number of first-degree relatives (mothers, sisters, or daughters) with breast cancer, a history of benign biopsy, age during delivery of a first child, and age at the start of menstuation. The women in STAR will receive either 20 mg of tamoxifen or 60 mg of Evista daily. We will know a lot more about whether Evista offers protection against breast cancer after this study is completed.

10

Take Charge of Your Health

Quick Fact: You have the right to expect considerate and respectful care from your doctor.

The patient in this case study is you, the reader. You may be in your twenties and in perfect health, in your forties and entering perimenopause, a symptom-free woman age 55 who has successfully made the transition to menopause, or a woman age 65 with osteoporosis. Whatever your age, the most important step any woman can take in staying healthy is taking charge of her health. Eating right, exercising, and not smoking or stopping smoking are just the initial steps. You need to be committed to feeling good and working with a responsive doctor in order to take a proactive, preventive approach to your health and body. Being informed, being responsible, and being part of your health care team will help keep you in charge.

You have learned a lot in this book about osteoporosis and Evista. You are now more informed about what causes osteoporosis and what you can do to avoid this bone-weakening disease and keep your bones healthy and strong for a lifetime. One of the reasons that osteoporosis has reached almost epidemic proportions in this country is because many women simply do not have the facts or are unaware of the need for prevention. Some think that osteoporosis is simply a natural and inevitable part of aging, while others think that it can never happen to them. Both views are mistaken. By educating yourself about osteoporosis and medications such as Evista you have taken a very important step. You should also share this knowledge with friends and loved ones to make sure that the women in your life learn how to fight this potentially disabling condition. As you saw in Chapter 2, it is never too early to do something about osteoporosis.

This book is not a substitute for professional medical care. But you can use the knowledge you have gained from this book to make informed and intelligent decisions about your health care and to forge a meaningful and lasting health-care partnership with your doctor. In my experience, informed patients usually get the best care. An informed patient is a woman who takes the time to find out as much as she can about her own health and the doctors who treat her. I enjoy treating women who care enough to educate themselves about the condition they are being treated for and who ask me intelligent questions about their care. A doctor who takes offense at thoughtful questioning is probably not the doctor with whom you will want to form a long-term partnership. You do not have to have a medical background in order to play an active part in caring for your health. After all, who cares more about your health than you?

By reading this book you have taken an important step in the right direction, but hopefully your efforts will not stop here. You could not have chosen a better time to take an active role in your health care. Never before has so much health information been available to the average woman in so many ways, especially with the appearance of health-related web sites on the Internet. This chapter can help. It provides tips on finding a doctor and getting the most out of the doctor-patient relationship. It is your starting point for tapping into the wealth of information available on osteoporosis, Evista, and menopause. Armed with this sort of information, you will be in a great position to make smart decisions about your health.

Q: What sort of doctor should I talk to about osteoporosis?

A: That is a good question. It is not quite as simple as finding a doctor with a degree in osteoporosis because there is no such thing. The truth is that a number of different doctors—doctors with different medical specialties—are qualified to treat women who have osteoporosis or who are concerned about preventing it. But it is possible to find a doctor whose practice is devoted largely to the treatment of women with osteoporosis. This doctor may be closer than you think. A good place to start is with your family doctor or gynecologist. Either of these doctors is familiar with your medical history and may be able to refer you to the doctors in your area who have the most experience treating women with osteoporosis. As a rule, family doctors do not have as much experience and expertise with osteoporosis, but they are at the front lines of osteoporosis prevention. As your guide during menopause, your gynecologist has more experience treating osteoporosis and other problems related to estrogen loss. In some cases you may wish to stay with your gynecologist, especially if your bones are healthy and your goal is to design a personal strategy of prevention. If you have been diagnosed with low bone density or have risk factors, you may benefit more from the experience of a doctor who devotes more time to this particular condition.

Q: So what type of doctor is best?

A: It is not really a case of one type of doctor being better than another. In addition to gynecologists, other doctors who commonly treat osteoporosis include endocrinologists, geriatricians, and rheumatologists. Endocrinologists specialize in diseases and problems of the endocrine system. As you saw in Chapter 1, estrogen and other hormones produced by glands in this system play an important role in bone health. Geriatricians are doctors who have received extra training in treating conditions associated with aging. Rheumatologists specialize in treating conditions that affect the joints, muscles, and bones. Internal medicine doctors, who treat diseases of the entire body, also treat women with osteoporosis. The goal is to find a doctor who has a lot of experience treating women with osteoporosis, because these doctors tend to be more up to date on the latest scientific research and medication. It is also important that you feel comfortable with the doctor who will be treating you.

Another good idea is to get in touch with an osteoporosis support group. You can do this by contacting some of the major hospitals or university medical centers in your area, since some of these institutions are associated with osteoporosis support groups. These groups can be enormously helpful in the sharing of information and support. The women in these groups may also be able to steer you toward the right doctor or away from the wrong ones. Talk to your regular doctor or contact some of the large hospitals in your area to find out about local osteoporosis support groups.

Q: Do you have any tips for choosing a doctor?

A: Choosing a doctor is a personal decision, but there are some general tips that may help. First of all, do not feel shy about shopping around for the right doctor. The health care industry is a service industry and you owe it to yourself to be an intelligent consumer. Finding a doctor who has experience treating osteoporosis is a major factor. But it is also important to find a doctor that you are comfortable with. The personal strategy crafted by you and your doctor to prevent or treat osteoporosis must last for a lifetime, so you want to choose an enduring doctor-patient partnership that will benefit you the most. To start off with, good communication skills are a must. Your doctor must have the ability to explain medical concepts in simple, understandable terms and be willing to take the time to make you understand. But a doctor must also be a good listener—someone who has a friendly manner and is attentive to your needs and concerns. Do not hesitate to check your doctor's credentials. Is your doctor board certified (a board-certified doctor has had extra training and passed an examination in a particular specialty)? Being board certified is a definite advantage. In addition to having extra training and expertise, studies show that board certified doctors are involved in fewer malpractice suits. If you have any doubts about a doctor's credentials, contact your state or ocal medical society for help. Find out what the doctor's seload is like and how much time in advance is needed schedule an appointment. Depending on your sched- you may wish to ask the doctor if after-hour or end appointments are available. Get your doctor's on preventing and treating osteoporosis. Find out the doctor feels about various treatment options discussed in this book. Some doctors discourage women from using certain medications while others evaluate treatment on a case-by-case basis. Talking to doctors with different points of view can be helpful.

Q: How can I get the most out of my doctor's visit?

A: First of all, find out as much as you can about osteoporosis and the different treatment options available. Your doctor will appreciate your initiative and you will find that having some background information is helpful when having discussions with your doctor. Make a list of questions to ask your doctor during your visit. Check off each question and do not move on to the next question until you are satisfied with the answer your doctor gives. Unfortunately, some women simply nod their heads and move on to the next question even though they do not fully understand what the doctor has said. You should not feel like you are wasting your doctor's time by asking questions and clarifying points that seem unclear. You have a right to understand all the implications of any treatment plan that you are considering.

Bringing a list of questions or discussion points to the doctor's office and anticipating what sort of information your doctor will ask of you during the visit shows your doctor that you are taking an active role in your own health care. Take some time to prepare yourself for questions that your doctor may ask about your medical history and that of your family, and bring your medical records with you. Running over a checklist, such as the Osteoporosis Risk Quiz presented in Chapter 2, makes it easier to answer your doctor's questions. This sort of preparedness helps to create a good partnership between you and your doctor. Ask your doctor if you can schedule an appointment just to talk. Too often women try to slip in their questions at the end of appointments when doctors are pressed for time and have other patients waiting.

Be honest with your doctor about your symptoms. You should never feel embarrassed about discussing any aspect of your health. Your doctor is there to help and your health is too important to jeopardize. If you have trouble recalling all your symptoms or any changes in your health, keep a health diary at home. Record basic facts about your symptoms or any changes, for better or worse, in your condition. This way you can present your doctor with an accurate picture of your health even when several months pass between visits. Doctors often have pamphlets or other helpful literature. Take this literature home with you and read it thoroughly. If you have questions about what you have read, write them down for your next visit. Do not depend on your memory. It is also important to let your doctor know when you are concerned about something. Doctors cannot read minds. If you do not emphasize your concerns, your doctor may not know that they are important to you.

Q: Do I have rights as a patient?

A: You certainly do. The foundation of a productive relationship between you and your doctor is based on mutual trust. You have the right to expect a certain level of care from your doctor. If you do not feel like you are receiving that level of care, you should not be shy about voicing your concerns to your doctor or switching to another practice. The Patient Bill of Rights adopted by the American Hospital Association (AHA) more than 20 years ago (and revised in 1992) explains the rights that you are entitled to as a patient. Some of these rights are listed below. You can get a full copy of the Patient Bill of Rights from the AHA—the contact information for this organization appears later in the chapter.

- You have the right to considerate and respectful care.
- You have the right to receive easy-to-understand information about your condition and any possible treatments from your doctor.
- You have the right to know the names and roles of the people treating you.
- You have the right to request from your doctor information about possible procedures or treatments and the risks involved, the possible length of recuperation, and the reasonable medical alternatives and their risks and possible benefits.
- You have the right to know the immediate and long-term financial implications of treatment choices, to the extent that they may be known.
- You have the right to consent to or to refuse a treatment to the extent permitted by law and to be informed of the medical consequences of this action. If you refuse a recommended treatment, you will receive other needed and available care.
- You have the right to privacy. Your doctor and other health professionals who care for you will protect your privacy as much as possible.
- You have the right to expect that treatment records are confidential unless you have given permission to release information or reporting is required by law. When the hospital release records to others, such as insurers, it emphasizes that the records are confidential.

- You have the right to review your medical records and to have the information explained if necessary, except when restricted by law.

Q: I am considering trying an alternative therapy to help ease my menopausal symptoms, but I am afraid to mention this to my doctor because I do not think my doctor will approve. Is there any harm in this?

A: There could be. Despite the fact that they are often derived from plants, these remedies sometimes have powerful effects that mimic those of natural hormones or prescription medications. For this reason, you should always discuss any of these therapies with a doctor before using it, especially if you are taking Evista or other prescription medication or have an existing medical condition. Your doctor may be more understanding than you think. Even if your doctor is opposed to the idea, it is worth hearing your doctor's professional point of view. Keep in mind that the safety and effectiveness of these remedies are largely unregulated by the federal government, so it makes sense to discuss your use of these products with your doctor, who knows your medical history and may be familiar with the latest scientific thinking regarding the therapy that you are using. Whether or not you decide to use an alternative therapy is up to you. If you decide to use one of these therapies, you may need some advice on the proper form and dosage to take. This is yet another good reason to talk to your doctor or a doctor who has experience with unconventional therapies before you experiment with them, and it is also a good reason to have an open-minded doctor who will consider different types of treatments. See later in this chapter for a listing of organizations that can provide more information on alternative therapies and that can help put you in touch with a doctor in your area who prescribes them.

Q: How can I find more information about osteoporosis or Evista?

A: There are many ways to go about it. Once you get tuned in to the idea of looking for health information, you may be surprised to find that there are sources of information all around you. This information can be found in books, newspapers, on television and the radio, and in medical journals. The Internet is also a great resource. One of the simplest ways to stay in touch with what is going on in the world of medicinc is to get in the daily habit of reading a major newspaper or news magazine or watching the news on TV. Health issues are big news these days. It is hard to pick up the paper or turn on the TV news without hearing about the latest findings on a new medication or disease. Many newspapers have special sections devoted to health and many television programs have medical correspondents who report regularly on health news. The results of major medical studies often make the news as well. But be cautious in interpreting what you see on television; often the information is not analyzed well or is sensationalized. There are numerous organizations and associations that provide information or support about osteoporosis. Organizations that provide information on menopause often have facts on osteoporosis and other problems associated with menopause.

Q: What sort of health information can I find on the Internet?

A: The answer is almost every kind. And you do not need to be an expert web surfer to access this vast resource.

Many of the organizations listed below have web sites on the Internet. These sites post information and often provide links to other areas of interest including online support groups. Anyone with access to the Internet can download information on osteoporosis, Evista and other osteoporosis medications, and menopause. Online sites can also provide a network of support and encouragement in the form of newsgroups and chat rooms. Newsgroups are areas in which people provide information and answer questions. In a chat room, you can participate in an ongoing, real-time group conversation on just about any subject. Search engines, such as Metacrawler, Altavista, Excite, WebCrawler, and Yahoo, make it possible to do Internet searches on specific topics. Once in a search engine, you can use osteoporosis-related search words in order to find relevant web sites. But caution is also necessary when using the Internet as a source for medical knowledge. While many legitimate organizations post information on the Internet, there are no guarantees that all the facts and recommendations that you find there will be sound. You may also find yourself the victim of a few sales pitches. It is always best to discuss what you discover on the Internet with your doctor.

Organizations That Provide Information or Support

American Academy of Family Physicians (AAFP)
8880 Ward Parkway
Kansas City, MO 64114
(816) 333-9700
http://www.aafp.org

The AAFP is a national, nonprofit medical association of more than 84,000 family doctors, family practice residents, and medical students. This web site has thousands of pages of health information, most of which can be downloaded by the public.

American Association of Clinical Endocrinologists (AACE)
1000 Riverside Avenue
Suite 205
Jacksonville, FL 32204
(904) 353-7878
http://www.aace.com/org/contact.html

The AACE is a professional medical organization devoted to the field of clinical endocrinology. If you are looking for an endocrinologist, you can use the online membership directory at this site to search by location and area of specialization. You will also find abstracts from the medical journal *Endocrine Practice* at this site.

American Association of Sex Educators, Counselors, and Therapists
Post Office Box 238
Mount Vernon, IA 52314
(319) 895-8407
http://www.aasect.org

The American Association of Sex Educators, Counselors, and Therapists (AASECT) is a not-for-profit professional organization that certifies sexual health practitioners and provides information about sexuality and sexual behavior. Information about the AASECT, its work, and related sites is available on the association's web site.

American Cancer Society (ACS)
1599 Clifton Road NE
Atlanta, GA 30329
(800) ACS-2345
http://www.cancer.org

The ACS provides up-to-date and comprehensive cancer information, including facts on alternative therapies. Much of this information is available on the web site.

American College of Obstetricians and Gynecologists (ACOG)
Office of Public Information
409 12th Street Southwest
Washington, DC 20024
(202) 484-3321
http://www.acog.com

Founded more than 45 years ago, ACOG is an association of than 37,000 physicians specializing in ob/gyn care. You will find patient information at this site and information on issues in women's health care.

American College of Rheumatology (ACR)
1800 Century Place
Suite 250
Atlanta, GA 30345
(404) 633-3777
http://www.rheumatology.org/index.html

The ACR is an organization of doctors, health professionals, and scientists that focuses on the care of people with arthritis and rheumatic and musculoskeletal diseases. You can use the Electronic Directory of Rheumatology at this site to help find a rheumatologist in your area. This site also provides links to other web sites related to rheumatic disorders. These links will take you to online journals, government agencies, and private organizations. You can do a literature search in ACR publications at this site as well.

The American Dietetic Association (ADA)
216 West Jackson Boulevard
Chicago, IL 60606
(312) 899-0040
http://www.eatright.org

The ADA promotes health and well-being by providing information on nutrition. You will find information on calcium and other minerals and vitamins at this site. You can also check out abstracts from the *Journal of the American Dietetic Association*, the official research publication of the ADA. You will also find information at this site on getting in touch with a registered dietitian.

American Heart Association (AHA)
7272 Greenville Avenue
Dallas, TX 75231
(800) AHA-USA-1
http://www.amhrt.org

This organization provides comprehensive information on heart disease and stroke, much of which is available on the web site.

American Hospital Association (AHA)
One North Franklin
Chicago, IL 60601
(312) 422-3000
http://www.aha.org

At the web site you can access articles from AHA publications. This site also provides health-care facts and figures, including a dictionary of selected health-care terms, and has an extensive list of links to other web sites that provide information on health care issues. You can also download a copy of the Patient Bill of Rights at this web site.

American Medical Association (AMA)
515 North State Street
Chicago, IL 60610
(312) 464-4818
http://www.ama-assn.org

Founded in 1847, the AMA is a professional association of doctors and medical students that provides authoritative health information for use by the public. The AMA publishes books and pamphlets and provides information on a variety of medical conditions on its web site. You can also use the AMA Physician Select feature to get the facts on more than 650,000 licensed doctors in the United States. The credentials of these doctors are verified for accuracy and authenticated by accrediting agencies, medical schools, residency training programs, licensing and certifying boards, and other sources. You can also access the *Journal of the American Medical Association* at this site.

American Medical Women's Association (AMWA)
801 North Fairfax Street
Suite 400
Alexandria, VA 22314
(703) 838-0500
http://www.amwa-doc.org/index.html

AMWA is an organization of more than 10,000 women doctors and medical students that emphasizes women's health concerns. This site provides information about a variety of different medical issues of interest to women. You can also access the *Journal of the American Medical Women's Association* at this site.

American Society for Reproductive Medicine (ASRM)
1209 Montgomery Highway
Birmingham, AL 35216
(205) 978-5000
http://www.asrm.org

Established in 1944, the ASRM focuses on reproductive medicine and biology. At this site you will find answers to frequently asked questions, patient education fact sheets and booklets, and information on ongoing medical studies.

Centers for Disease Control and Prevention (CDC)
1600 Clifton Road Northeast
Atlanta, GA 30333
(404) 639-3311
http://www.cdc.gov

As the nation's prevention agency, the CDC is responsible for promoting health and quality of life by preventing and controlling disease, injury, and disability. Among other things, the CDC conducts research on preventive medicine, develops and advocates public health policies, and promotes healthy behavior. The CDC is made up of 11 centers, institutes, and offices, including an Office on Women's Health.

Food and Drug Administration (FDA)
5600 Fisher's Lane

Rockville, MD 20857
(301) 827-2410
http://www.fda.gov

At this site you can access the FDA's Office of Women's Health. It provides information on the latest medications approved to treat women's health conditions and has other information on women's health. This site is a great place to find out more about medications—including new uses for FDA-approved medications—and the medication-approval process.

Harvard Health Publications
http://www.countway.harvard.edu/publications/Health_Publications/home.html

At this site you can access feature articles from the *Harvard Health Letter* newsletter and other periodicals from Harvard Health Publications. This site also features a question-and-answer section where you can get answers to a variety of health questions.

Healthfinder
http://www.healthfinder.org/default.htm

Launched in 1997, Healthfinder is a resource for health information from the federal government. It can lead you to online publications, clearinghouses, databases, web sites, and support and self-help groups, as well as to government agencies and nonprofit organizations that provide information to the public.

HERS Foundation
Hysterectomy Educational Resources and Services
422 Bryn Mawr Avenue

Bala Cynwyd, PA 19004
(610) 667-7757
http://www.ccon.com/hers

The HERS Foundation is an international nonprofit women's health education organization. It provides information about hysterectomy, its adverse effects, and alternative treatments. It provides free information by mail, telephone counseling by appointment, doctor referral for treatment options, referral to lawyers, litigation support, video and audio tapes, review of medical or surgical records, reading lists of suggested books and medical articles, and woman-to-woman networking. It also provides information on estrogen replacement therapy (ERT) and hormone replacement therapy (HRT).

Mayo Health Oasis
http://www.mayohealth.org/mayo/common/htm/index.htm

Updated every weekday, this site presents up-to-date information on the prevention and treatment of a wide variety of medical conditions from the doctors and scientists at the Mayo Clinic. This site has a Women's Center, sections on Alzheimer's disease as well as on diet and nutrition, and a Heart Center. You will also find information on medications at this site.

MEDLINE
http://www.nlm.nih.gov/databases/freemedl.html

At this site you can access a database of more than 9 million references to articles published in 3,800 biomedical journals. You can read abstracts of medical journal articles at this site. You can do searches by entering keywords such as "osteoporosis" or "raloxifene" (the generic name for Evista).

Menopause News
2074 Union Street
San Francisco, CA 94123
(800) 241-MENO
http://www.well.com/user/mnews/html/experts.htm

Menopause News is a newsletter founded in 1991 and devoted to issues related to menopause. You can check out sample articles on the web site and get other information on menopause.

Menopause Online
http://www.menopause-online.com

This site is devoted to providing women with up-to-date, easy-to-use information on menopause and menopause-related health concerns. You will find information here on ERT and HRT, osteoporosis and osteoporosis medications, and alternative therapies.

National Cancer Institute (NCI)
1-800-4-CANCER
http://www.nci.nih.gov

The NCI is a part of the National Institutes of Health (NIH), the main biomedical research agency of the federal government. The NCI coordinates the Natioanl Cancer Program, which conducts and supports research, the training of health professionals, and the education of the public about all aspects of cancer.

National Health Information Center (NHIC)
U.S. Department of Health and Human Services
Referral Specialist
P.O. Box 1133

Washington, DC 20013
(301) 565-4167
(800) 336-4797
http://nhic-nt.health.org

Formerly the National Health Information Clearinghouse, the NHIC was established in 1979 as a health information referral service. It can help guide you toward organizations that are best able to provide answers to your health questions. The NHIC also has a collection of health reference materials, journals, newsletters, and educational materials available for use by the public.

National Institute of Arthritis and Musculoskeletal and Skin Diseases (NIAMS)
National Institutes of Health
Bethesda, Maryland 20892-2350
(301) 496-4000
http://www.nih.gov/niams

NIAMS is a part of the NIH and provides information on arthritis and diseases of the musculoskeletal system and the skin. It offers fact sheets (including a fact sheet on hip replacement), brochures, and health statistics.

National Institute on Aging (NIA)
Post Office Box 8057
Gaithersburg, MD 20898
(800) 222-2225
http://www.nih.gov/nia

Part of the NIH, the NIA produces educational materials on a wide range of topics related to health and aging. Topics cover specific diseases and health conditions, treatments, and research. The materials are for use by the public and some are available online.

National Osteoporosis Foundation (NOF)
1150 17th Street Northwest
Suite 500
Washington, DC 20036
(202) 223-2226
http://www.nof.org

The NOF is often referred to as America's leading resource for people seeking up-to-date, medically sound information on the causes, prevention, detection, and treatment of osteoporosis. The NOF can provide you with useful information, support, and guidance.

National Women's Health Resource Center (NWHRC)
5255 Loughboro Road Northwest
Washington, DC 20016
(202) 537-4015
http://www.healthywomen.org/about.html

NWHRC, a nonprofit organization, is a national clearinghouse for information and resources about women's health. The stated purpose of the organization is to educate healthcare consumers and empower them to make intelligent decisions by providing easy-to-understand information and accessible services.

North American Menopause Society (NAMS)
University Hospitals
Department of Ob/Gyn
P.O. Box 94527
Cleveland, OH 44101

(216) 844-8748
http://www.menopause.org

NAMS is an organization of 2,000 doctors and other health care professionals from the United States, Canada, Mexico, and other countries around the world. Members include experts from medicine, anthropology, sociology, and psychology. The stated objective of NAMS is to provide accurate, unbiased information about all aspects of menopause.

Sexuality Information and Education Council of the
United States (SIECUS)
130 West 42nd Street
Suite 350
New York, NY 10036
(212) 819-9770
http://www.siecus.org

SIECUS is a 33-year-old nonprofit organization that provides information, promotes comprehensive education, and advocates the right of people to make responsible sexual choices. SIECUS publishes and distributes thousands of new and revised pamphlets, booklets, and bibliographies each year.

U.S. Department of Agriculture
14th and Independence Avenue, Southwest
Washington, D.C. 20250
(202) 720-2791
http://www.usda.gov

At this site you will find a wealth of information on health and nutrition and have access to federal health guidelines and links to related sites. Here you can download a copy of *Dietary Guidelines for Americans*, the federal government's statement of nutrition policy, formed by a group of scientific and medical professionals. This site also features the USDA Nutrient Database Search and has information on recommended daily allowances.

World Health Organization (WHO)
Regional Office for the Americas/Pan American Health Organization (AMRO/PAHO)
525 23rd Street Northwest
Washington, DC 20037
(202) 974-3000
http://www.who.org

This world-renowned organization provides fact sheets, publications, periodicals, and statements of WHO health policies. Some of this information can be downloaded at the web site.

Organizations That Provide Information Mainly on Alternative Therapies

The American Association of Naturopathic Physicians (AANP)
P.O. Box 20386
Seattle, WA 98102
(206) 323-7610
http://www.naturopathic.org

The AANP provides information on alternative therapies and the holistic approach to medicine. Holistic medicine emphasizes treating the whole person—physical, mental, emotional, and spiritual. You can use the search engine at this site to locate a licensed naturopathic doctor in your area who belongs to the AANP. You can also access the *Journal of Naturopathic Medicine* at this site.

The American Holistic Medical Association (AHMA)
4101 Lake Boone Trail, #201
Raleigh, NC 26707
(919) 787-5146
http://www.ahmaholistic.com

Founded in 1978, the AHMA is an organization of doctors and state-licensed holistically oriented practitioners such as chiropractors, naturopaths, nurses, and psychologists. At this site you will find information about holistic medicine and can access articles from *Holistic Medicine Magazine*.

The Herb Research Foundation (HRF)
1007 Pearl Street
Suite 200
Boulder, CO 80302
(303) 449-2265
http://www.herbs.org/index.html

The HRF is a nonprofit research and educational organization focusing on herbs and medicinal plants. The stated purpose of the HRF is to improve world health and well-being through herbs. This organization has more than 150,000 scientific articles in its botanical library. The HRF provides information on thousands of herbs. The HRF publishes a herb magazine called *HerbalGram*, the *Herb Research News* newsletter, and another magazine called *Herbs for Health.*

National Center for Homeopathy (NCH)
801 North Fairfax Street

Suite 306
Alexandria, VA 22314
(703) 548-7790
http://www.healthy.net/pan/pa/homeopathic/natcenhom

The stated purpose of the NCH is to promote health through homeopathy. It provides general information to the public about homeopathy and has a staff that answers more than 10,000 inquiries a year. The NCH conducts homeopathy classes for laypeople and health-care professionals. It publishes an educational publication called *Homeopathy Today* and offers a *Directory of Homeopathic Practitioners*, which provides information on practitioners, study groups, pharmacies, and resources. The NCF also has a library with one of the largest collections of homeopathic literature in the United States.

Books on Osteoporosis and Menopause

Before the Change: Taking Charge of Your Perimenopause, A. L. Gittleman. Harper, 1998.

Better Bones, Better Body, S. E. Brown and P. Herman. Keats, 1996.

Bone-Loading: Exercises for Osteoporosis, A. Simkin and J. Ayalon. Trafalgar Square, 1997.

Controlling Hormones Naturally: My Journey for Solutions to PMS, Menopause and Osteoporosis with Wild Yam, M. Bonk, L. M. Aesoph, and L. K. Fraser. MB Publishers, 1996.

Dr. Susan Love's Hormone Book: Making Informed Choices about Menopause, S. M. Love. Random House, 1998.

Eating Well, Living Well with Osteoporosis: Dietary Approaches to Healthy Living, C. W. Bales, T. Schusterman, and P. H. Lin. Viking, 1996.

The Estrogen Alternative: Natural Hormone Therapy with Botanical Progesterone, R. Martin and J. Gerstung. Inner Traditions, 1998.

Estrogen: Answers to All Your Questions About Hormone Replacement Therapy and Natural Alternatives, M. Stolar. Avon, 1997.

Food and Our Bones, A. Colbin. Plume, 1998.

Healthy Bones: What You Should Know about Osteoporosis, N. Appleton. Avery, 1997.

Holistic Menopause, J. Hall. Findhorn, 1998.

How to Fight Osteoporosis and Win!: The Miracle of Microcrystalline Hydroxyapitite (Mchc), B.M. Ley. BL Publications, 1996.

I Love Menopause Because . . ., J. S. Ben-Kiki and R. S. Herman. Andrews and McMeel, 1998.

I'm Too Young to Get Old: Health Care for Women after Forty, J. Reichman. Random House, 1998.

Keys to Understanding Osteoporosis, J. Rozek. Barron's, 1992.

The Menopause, S. Brewer. Thorsons, 1997.

Menopause: A Gentle, Natural Approach, E. C. Ryneveld. Llewellyn, 1998.

Menopause: A Guide to Health and Happiness, J. E. Huston. Facts On File, 1998.

Menopause and Madness: The Truth about Estrogen and Mental Health, M. Lawrence and C. Schillig. Andrews McMeel, 1998.

Menopause and Osteoporosis: Taking Control of Your Life Change, L. R. Page. Healthy Healing, 1998.

Menopause Madness, P. Ross. Fireside, 1998.

The Menopause Manager: A Safe Path for a Natural Change, M. A. Mayo and J. L. Mayo. Fleming H. Revell, 1997.

The Menopause SourceBook, G. Henkel. Lowell House, 1998.

The Natural Estrogen Book: A Natural Treatment for the Symptoms of Menopause, L. Liew. Simon and Schuster Australia, 1998.

Natural Woman, Natural Menopause, M. Laux. Harper-Collins, 1998.

No More Hot Flashes . . . and Even More Good News, P. W. Budoff. Warner, 1998.

One Hundred and Fifty Most Asked Questions about Osteoporosis: What Women Really Want to Know, R. S. Jacobowitz. William Morrow, 1996.

Osteoporosis, D. Lee. Woodland, 1997.

Osteoporosis: A Natural Approach to Prevention, W. Stephens. Westeron Stephens III, 1995.

The Osteoporosis Cure: Reverse the Crippling Effects with New Treatments, H. McIlwain. Avon, 1998.

The Osteoporosis Handbook, S. L. Bonnick. Taylor, 1997.

Osteoporosis: How to Make Your Bones Last a Lifetime, C. S. Lyon and C. E. Sutton. Soho, 1994.

Osteoporosis—Questions and Answers, J. Stevenson and M. C. Ellerington. Merit, 1994.

Outsmarting the Mid-Life Fat Cell: The Foolproof Weight Control Program Designed Specifically for Menopause, D. Waterhouse. Hyperion, 1998.

Passage to Power: Natural Menopause Revolution, L. Kenton. Hay House, 1998.

The Pause: Positive Approaches to Menopause, L. G. Barbach. Signature, 1998.

The Perimenopause Handbook: What Every Woman Needs to Know about the Years before Menopause, C. A. Turkington. Contemporary, 1998.

Permanent Remissions: Life-Extending Diet Strategies That Can Help Prevent and Reverse Cancer, Heart Disease, Diabetes, and Osteoporosis, R. Haas. Pocket, 1997.

Power of Perimenopause, S. D. Bender. Harmony, 1998.

Preventing and Reversing Osteoporosis: Every Woman's Essential Guide, A. R. Gaby. Prima, 1995.

Research and Recipes on Dementia, Heart Disease, Osteoporosis and Cancer, R. C. Fisher. Warren H. Green, 1997.

Save Your Bones!: High Calcium, Low Calorie Recipes for the Family, L. Goulder. Triad, 1998.

The Silent Passage: Menopause, G. Sheehy. Pocket, 1998.

Solved: The Riddle of Osteoporosis, S. Langer and J. F. Scheer. Keats, 1997.

Super Calcium Miracle: Finally . . . a Proven Program to Help Reduce the Risk of Osteoporosis, M. Andon. Prima, 1998.

Trouble-Free Menopause: Manage Your Symptoms and Your Weight, J. E. Marshel. Avon, 1998.

What Every Woman Needs to Know about Menopause: The Years Before, During and After, M. J. Minkin and C. V. Wright. Yale University, 1997.

Winning with Osteoporosis, H. H. McElwain, D. F. Bruce, J. C. Silverfield, and M. C. Burnette. John Wiley and Sons, 1994.

Woman Doctor's Guide to Osteoporosis: Essential Facts and Up-to-the-Minute Information on the Prevention, Treatment and Reversal of Bone Loss, Y. Sherrer and R. K. Levinson. Hyperion, 1994.

Women at the Change: The Intelligent Woman's Guide to Menopause, M. S. Compton. Llewellyn, 1998.

Women, Hormones and the Menstrual Cycle: Herbal and Medical Solutions from Adolescence to Menopause, R. Trickey. Allen and Unwin, 1998.

Your Menopause: Real Information You Can Use, R. J. Shields. CEPI, 1997.

Glossary

acupuncture: the insertion of very thin needles into certain areas of the body, used to treat illnesses and to relieve stress or pain.

adrenal glands: glands of the endocrine system that produce hormones such as cortisone and androgen.

aerobic exercise: exercise that makes the heart and lungs work harder to meet the increased oxygen demands of the body; aerobic exercise helps to condition the heart and may also increase HDL cholesterol levels in some women.

alendronate: a bone-building osteoporosis medication sold under the brand name Fosamax.

amenorrhea: an abnormal missing of menstrual periods.

androgens: important male sex hormones found in small amounts in women and sometimes added to estrogen replacement therapy.

angina: a chronic condition characterized by brief episodes of chest pain or shortness of breath.

anorexia nervosa: a dangerous obsession with thinness, usually affecting young women, that goes beyond normal dieting; anorexics have a distorted body image and an abnormal need to control food.

atherosclerosis: hardening of the arteries.

biochemical marker: a substance found in blood or urine that gives doctors clues to processes going on inside the body; sometimes used to monitor the bone-remodeling process.

biofeedback training: a behavior-modification technique often used to manage stress; in biofeedback training, a person is given information about involuntary body functions (such as blood pressure or heart rate) with the hope that the person will gain voluntary control of those body functions.

bone density: the amount of mineral in any given volume of bone.

bone density test: a medical test used to measure the strength of the bones.

bone loss: a reduction in bone density.

bone mass: the total amount of bone in the skeleton; the phrases *bone density* and *bone mass* are often used interchangeably in osteoporosis literature.

bone mineral density (BMD): a measurement of the amount of mineral found in bone; the BMD measurement is obtained by a bone density test.

bone remodeling: the process by which bones are broken down (by osteoclast cells) and rebuilt (by osteoblast cells) over a lifetime.

calcitonin: a hormone produced in the thyroid gland that helps prevent bone loss and is used in synthetic form as a bone-building medication sold under the brand names Miacalcin and Calcimar.

calcium: a mineral that acts as an important building block of bone and is used by the body for proper functioning of organs and muscles.

cancer: an unrestrained growth of abnormal cells, often in the form of a tumor, that invades and destroys healthy tissue.

cardiovascular system: the system responsible for circulating blood throughout the body. Composed mainly of the heart and blood vessels.

chemotherapy: the use of certain medications to treat infections or cancer.

cholesterol: a soft, fatty substance made by the body and also found in foods that come from animals.

compression fracture: a fracture of a vertebra.

cortical bone: the hard and compact bone tissue making up 85% of all bone in your body.

corticosteroid: hormones produced by the adrenal gland and used in synthetic form to treat inflammation and suppress autoimmune responses and used in the treatment of various disorders.

dementia: a gradual decline in mental ability usually caused by a brain disease such as Alzheimer's disease.

diuretics: agents that increase urination.

dowager's hump: a condition in which the spine is bent forward due to fractured vertebrae, causing a stooped posture; also called kyphosis.

dual energy X-ray absorptiometry (DEXA): a procedure that uses very low levels of radiation to measure bone density.

early menopause: menopause that occurs before age 40.

edema: swelling, usually in the legs and ankles but sometimes in other parts of the body as well, due to fluid retention.

endocrine system: a complex biological network composed of organs and glands that secrete hormones to other areas of the body in order to regulate a variety of body functions; in women this network includes the ovaries, thyroid gland, pituitary gland, adrenal glands, pancreas, thymus, and hypothalamus.

endocrinologist: a doctor who specializes in the diagnosis and treatment of disorders of the endocrine system.

estradiol: the main estrogen; produced by the ovaries, estradiol operates from puberty to menopause and is measured by doctors to determine estrogen levels.

estrogen: an important female sex hormone, made primarily in the ovaries, that helps to keep bones healthy and strong and has a variety of effects on other body functions.

estrogen receptors: proteins on the surfaces of cells that bind with estrogen; once produced by an organ or gland, estrogen is sent through the bloodstream to a specific receptor on another organ or gland (into which it fits as does a key into a lock), where it either turns on or turns off—or speeds up or slows down—activity at the site.

estrogen replacement therapy (ERT): a medication used to replace estrogen in menopausal and postmenopausal women.

Evista® (raloxifene): a bone-building medication, belonging to the selective estrogen receptor modulator (SERM) class, approved by the Food and Drug Administration in 1997 for osteoporosis.

follicle-stimulating hormone (FSH): a hormone produced by the pituitary gland that stimulates estrogen secretion and the growth of follicles in the ovary.

fracture: a break in a bone.

fracture threshold: a phrase used by doctors to describe a bone density measurement that is dangerously low; if bone density falls just below the fracture threshold, the risk of fracturing a bone is about two times that of a woman who has healthy bones.

gland: a cell (or group of cells) or an organ that produces substances (such as hormones) used by the body.

heart attack: a degeneration of the heart muscle that results from inadequate blood supply to the area.

high density lipoprotein (HDL): a protein that transports cholesterol away from the arteries and back to the liver, where it is passed from the body or used to make other substances; also called "good" cholesterol.

hormone: a chemical message carrier produced by an organ or gland that helps to regulate the healthy functioning of the body.

hormone replacement therapy (HRT): a medication in which a form of progesterone is added to estrogen replacement therapy in order to cut the risk of cancer of the uterus associated with estrogen replacement therapy alone.

hot flash: a temporary sensation of heat in the face, neck, and chest, often accompanied by sweating and chills, that results from low estrogen levels.

hypothalamus: the part of the brain above the pituitary gland that regulates many body functions such as body temperature, sleep, and appetite.

hysterectomy: a surgical procedure in which the entire uterus is removed.

insomnia: difficulty falling or staying asleep.

lactose intolerance: a condition in which dairy products are not easily digested; it is important for women with lactose intolerance to get calcium from nondairy sources or calcium supplements.

libido: sexual drive or desire.

ligaments: the tissues that hold together the joints of bones.

lipoprotein: a substance that transports fats in the blood.

low-density lipoprotein (LDL): a protein that tends to deposit cholesterol onto the walls of the arteries, where it may build up and form plaque; also called "bad" cholesterol.

luteinizing hormone (LH): a hormone produced by the pituitary gland that acts with FSH to stimulate ovulation and the making of androgen and progesterone.

magnesium: a mineral that is essential for many body functions including the formation of bones.

mammogram: an X ray of the breast.

menopause: the day on which menstrual periods have stopped for a period of one year, occurring around age 50; this term is also used to refer to the entire process during which the ovaries slow down and finally cease producing estrogen.

metastasis: the spread of cancerous cells from one region of the body to another.

mineral: an inorganic substance, found in food and dietary supplements, that is essential to the healthy functioning of the body.

monounsaturated fat: a type of unsaturated fat that may help to reduce blood cholesterol levels.

musculoskeletal system: the muscles, ligaments, tendons, and bones of the human body.

osteoblasts: the cells that remove calcium and other minerals from the blood and add them to bone, making bone stronger.

osteoclasts: the cells that remove calcium and other minerals from bone and send them back into the blood, making bone weaker.

osteoporosis: an age-related gradual weakening of the bones that causes them to become more fragile and vulnerable to potentially debilitating fractures.

ovary: the female reproductive organ that produces eggs; the ovaries are where most of a women's estrogen is made.

parathyroid hormone: a hormone, made in small glands located in the neck, that regulates the levels of calcium in the blood; when calcium blood levels are low, parathyroid hormone signals the osteoclasts to work harder to remove bone.

peak bone density: the state in which your bones are at their strongest.

perimenopausal: a term meaning "around the time of menopause"; perimenopause is usually accompanied by irregular periods and sometimes other menopausal symptoms.

pituitary gland: a tiny gland located at the base of the brain that controls hormone production in other endocrine glands.

placebo: a sugar pill; used mainly in controlled experiments to test the efficacy of another substance (usually a medication).

plaque: a buildup of cholesterol and other substances (including calcium) in the lining of an artery.

polyunsaturated fat: a type of unsaturated fat that may help to reduce blood cholesterol levels.

postmenopausal: a term referring to a woman who has completed menopause.

primary osteoporosis: osteoporosis that is not caused by the effects of a disease or medication.

progesterone: a female sex hormone made by the ovaries, primarily responsible for preparing the uterus for the fertilized egg and for the growth and development of the fetus, and sometimes added to estrogen replacement therapy to cut the risk of cancer of the uterus.

progestin: a synthetic form of progesterone used in HRT.

protein: a substance, made up of amino acids, which helps to grow and repair tissue in the body and also forms the basis for new bone.

radiation: a type of energy found in X rays and ultraviolet light.

saturated fat: a type of fat, found mainly in foods that come from animals and in certain vegetable oils, that can raise your blood cholesterol levels.

secondary osteoporosis: osteoporosis caused by the effects of a disease or medication.

selective estrogen receptor modulators (SERMs): a class of medications that mimic the effects of estrogen in certain parts of the body but not in others.

sodium: a mineral that plays a role in the body's water balance, heart rhythm, nerve impulses, and muscle contraction; present in table salt (sodium chloride).

sodium fluoride: the fluoride found in toothpaste and tap water; sodium fluoride is being studied as a potential osteoporosis medication.

stroke: damage to part of the brain caused by lack of blood supply (due to a blockage in an artery) or the rupturing of a blood vessel.

surgical menopause: an onset of menopause caused by the surgical removal of the ovaries.

testosterone: a male sex hormone produced in the testes.

thrombosis: a blood clot.

trabecular bone: the spongelike type of bone making up 15% of all bone in the body.

type 1 osteoporosis: osteoporosis that occurs primarily due to loss of estrogen during menopause; also called postmenopausal osteoporosis.

type 2 osteoporosis: osteoporosis affecting both men and women over age 70; also called senile osteoporosis.

unsaturated fat: a type of fat that may have a healthy effect on the heart when used in moderation; monounsaturated fat and polyunsaturated fat are both unsaturated fats.

urinary tract: the structures in the body responsible for the production and release of urine; the urinary tract includes the kidneys, ureters, bladder, and urethra.

vagina: the muscular passage connecting the uterus with the outside of the body—a component of the female reproductive system.

vertebra: any one of the 33 bones that make up the spine.

vitamin: one of a group of organic substances, found in food or dietary supplements, that are essential to the healthy functioning and proper development of the body.

vitamin D: a vitamin that helps the body use calcium better; vitamin D is manufactured by the body in response to direct sunlight and is also found in certain foods.

weight-bearing exercise: exercise that puts stress on muscle and bone; weight-bearing exercises help build up bone density and prevent the bones from becoming brittle.

Index

AACE, *see* American Association of Clinical Endocrinologists (AACE)
AAFP, *see* American Academy of Family Physicians (AAFP)
AANP, *see* American Association of Naturopathic Physicians (AANP)
ACOG, *see* American College of Obstetricians and Gynecologists (ACOG)
ACR, *see* American College of Rheumatology (ACR)
ACS, *see* American Cancer Society (ACS)
Acupuncture, 42
ADA, *see* American Dietetic Association (ADA)
Adrenal hormones, 26
AHA, *see* American Heart Association (AHA)
AHMA, *see* American Holistic Medical Association (AHMA)
Alcohol
  bones and, 137
  calcium and, 137
  heart disease and, 137, 158
  sleeping difficulties and, 98
Alcoholism
  osteoporosis and, 16–17, 25
  vitamin D absorption, 17, 25, 137
Alendronate, 39, 63, 73, 110, 123–24
  side effects, 124
Alternative therapies
  Alzheimer's disease and, 107–8
  anxiety and, 104
  Evista, while taking, 89–90
  hot flashes and, 93–95
  informational sources, 189–91
  moodiness and, 104
  physicians and, 175
  sleeping difficulties and, 99
  vaginal dryness and, 103
Alzheimer's disease
  alternative therapies for, 107–8
  Aricept and, 107
  Cognex and, 107
  Coumadin and, 108
  estrogen replacement therapy (ERT) and, *see* Estrogen replacement therapy (ERT)
  Ginkgo biloba and, 108
  Panwarfin and, 108
  Sofarin and, 108
  vitamin E and, 108
  Warfarin and, 108

AMA, *see* American Medical Association (AMA)
American Academy of Family Physicians (AAFP), 177
American Association of Clinical Endocrinologists (AACE), 178
American Association of Naturopathic Physicians (AANP), 189
American Association of Sex Educators, Counselors, and Therapists, 178
American Cancer Society (ACS), 179
American College of Obstetricians and Gynecologists (ACOG), 179
American College of Rheumatology (ACR), 179
American Dietetic Association (ADA), 180
American Heart Association (AHA), 180
American Holistic Medical Association (AHMA), 190
American Hospital Association (AHA), 180
American Medical Association (AMA), 181
American Medical Women's Association (AMWA), 181
American Society for Reproductive Medicine (ASRM), 182
Ampicillin, Evista and, 82
AMWA, *see* American Medical Women's Association (AMWA)
Androgen
  disadvantages of, 118
  estrogen replacement therapy (ERT) combined with, 117–18
Anorexia nervosa, 27–28
Antibiotics, Evista and, 83
Anxiety, 103
  alternative therapies for, 104
Aricept, Alzheimer's disease and, 107
Arthritis, 49
ASRM, *see* American Society for Reproductive Medicine (ASRM)
Atromid-S, Evista and, 82

Bellergal, 96
Bisphosphonates, 126
Black cohosh, hot flashes and, 94–95
Blood clots
  estrogen replacement therapy (ERT) and, 120
  Evista and, *see* Evista
  warning signs, 85
BMD, *see* Bone mineral density (BMD)
Bone density test, 32
Bone mineral density (BMD), 32
  fracture threshold, 36–37
Bones
  alcohol and, 137
  calcium and, 6–7
  composition of, 5–6
  cortical, 6
  trabecular, 6
  types of, 6
Breast cancer, 158–63
  Breast Cancer Prevention Trial (BCPT), 164
  defined, 158
  estrogen replacement therapy (ERT) and, *see* Estrogen replacement therapy (ERT)
  Evista, *see* Evista
  mammograms, 160–61
  self-examination, 161–62
  statistics on, 148, 160
  symptoms of, 160
  tamoxifen and, 163–64

Caffeine
  Evista and, 78
  osteoporosis and, 18, 25–26, 138
  sleeping difficulties and, 98
Calcimar, 40, 110, 126
Calcitonin, 12, 40, 110
  defined, 125
Calcitrol, 126
Calcium
  alcohol and, 137
  bones and, 6–7
  deficiency, 17
  importance of, 131
  sources of, 24, 133
  supplements, 23, 64, 77, 111, 134
CDC, *see* Centers for Disease Control and Prevention (CDC)
Centers for Disease Control and Prevention (CDC), 182
CHF, *see* Congestive heart failure (CHF)
Cholesterol
  coronary heart disease (CHD), risk factor for, 152
  defined, 152
  fats and, 154–55
  LDL, HDL differentiated from, 153–54
Cholestyramine, Evista and, 82
Clofibrate, Evista and, 82
Cognex, Alzheimer's disease and, 107
Collagen, 12
Compression fractures, 13, 46–47
  exercise and, 141
Computed tomography (CT), 34, 35
Congestive heart failure (CHF), 149
  Evista and, 79
Coronary heart disease (CHD), 148–49
  cholesterol, risk factor in, 152
Cortical bone, 6
Coumadin
  Alzheimer's disease and, 108
  Evista and, 82
CT, *see* Computed tomography (CT)
Cushing syndrome, 18

D-amp, Evista and, 82
Depression, 103
  warning signs, 105
DEXA, *see* Dual energy X-ray absorptiometry (DEXA)
Diabetes, 18
Diazoxide, Evista and, 83
Didronel, 126
Diet, importance of healthy, 130
  bone strength and, 135
  heart disease and, 156
Dilantin, 18
Dowager's hump, 13, 47
DPA, *see* Dual photon absorptiometry (DPA)
Dual energy X-ray absorptiometry (DEXA), 34, 36, 75
Dual photon absorptiometry (DPA), 34, 36

Echinacea, 101
Endocrine system, 170
ERT, *see* Estrogen replacement therapy (ERT)
Estratest, 117
Estrogen
  creams, 113–14
  hormones, effects on other, 12
  memory loss and, 106
  patches, 113–14
  pills, 113–14
Estrogen replacement therapy (ERT), 61, 112
  Alzheimer's disease and, 68, 107, 110, 123
  androgen combined with, 117–18
  benefits of, 38

(ERT) (*continued*)
blood clots and, 120
breast cancer and, 38, 68, 118–19, 122–23
cancer and, 110
disadvantages of, 115
Evista distinguished from, 67–68, 112–13, 120–23
Evista, interactions with, 82
heart disease and, 110, 116–17
high-density lipoprotein (HDL), affect on, 116–17
hot flashes and, 68, 89, 115, 122
low density lipoprotein (LDL), affect on, 116–17
menopausal symptoms and, 110, 115, 122
night sweats and, 68, 89
progesterone and, 115
risk factors, 38
side effects, 119–20, 121
uterine cancer and, 38, 68, 118–19, 122–23
vaginal dryness and, 68, 89
Estrogen-androgen therapy, 117, 122
Etidronate, 126
Evista, 39, 62–86, 147
allergic reactions to, 80
alternative therapies and, 89–90
blood clots and, 66, 73, 79, 84
body, affects on, 67
breast cancer and, 63, 79, 122–23, 147, 161
caffeine and, 78
calcium supplements and, 64, 77
cautions, 85
cirrhosis, danger associated with, 80
effectiveness of, 64–65, 73, 74–76
estrogen replacement therapy (ERT) distinguished from, 67–68, 112–13, 120–23
estrogen replacement therapy (ERT), interactions with, 82
exercise and, 77–78
fractures, prevention of, 65
heart disease and, 63, 121–22, 150–52
hot flashes and, 65, 74, 84, 89, 122
informational sources, 176–77
ingredients in, 81
medications, interactions with other, 82–83
menopausal symptoms, effect on, 89, 122
night sweats and, 89
osteoporosis, effectiveness on, 120
ovarian cancer and, 66–67
over-the-counter medications and, 74, 80, 89
safety of, 69–70, 72, 78
side effects, 73, 79–80, 121
smoking and, 78, 80
uterine cancer and, 79, 122–23
vitamin D supplements and, 64, 77
who should not take it, 66, 79–80
Exercise, 130
benefits of, 139–40
Evista and, 77–78
falls, prevention of, 50, 57–58
flexion, 141
hot flashes and, 92–93
osteoporosis and, 18, 24–25, 141
sleeping difficulties and, 98
weight-bearing, 24–25

Falls, 47–51
causes of, 48–49
exercise and, 50, 57–58
indoors, prevention techniques, 51–56
medications, side effects of, 49–50

outdoors, prevention techniques, 56–57
Fatigue, Korean ginseng and, 100
FDA, *see* Food and Drug Administration (FDA)
Flexion exercise, 141
Food and Drug Administration (FDA), 182
Food Guide Pyramid, 138–39, 140
Forgetfulness, *see* Memory loss
Fosamax, *see* Alendronate
Fracture threshold, 36
Fractures
compression, *see* Compression fractures
Evista and, 65
hip, 13, 43–46
side effects, 65–66
vertebral, 46–47
wrist, 47
Framingham Heart Study, 148

Ginkgo biloba, 90
Alzheimer's disease and, 108
memory loss and, 106
Ginseng, *see* Korean ginseng
Goldenseal, vaginal dryness and, 103
Growth factors, 126

Harvard Health Publications, 183
Hawthorn, memory loss and, 106
HDL, *see* High-density lipoprotein (HDL)
Healthfinder, 183
Heart disease
alcohol and, 137, 158
congestive heart failure (CHF), 79, 149
coronary heart disease (CHD), 148–49, 152
estrogen replacement therapy (ERT) and, 110, 116–117
Evista and, *see* Evista
Framingham Heart Study, 148
menopause and, 148
preventive measures, 156–158
smoking and, 156
statistics on, 148
Herb Research Foundation (HRF), 190
HERS Foundation, 183
High-density lipoprotein (HDL)
estrogen replacement therapy (ERT) affect on, 116–17
Evista's affect on, 151
Hip fractures, 13, 43–46
Hormone replacement therapy (HRT), *see* Estrogen replacement therapy (ERT)
Hot flashes, 30
alternative therapies for, 93–95
Bellergal and, 96
causes of, 90–92
estrogen replacement therapy (ERT) and, *see* Estrogen replacement therapy (ERT)
Evista and, *see* Evista
exercise and, 92–93
medications for, 96
soy and, 95
triggers, 91–92
HRF, *see* Herb Research Foundation (HRF)
HRT, *see* Estrogen replacement therapy (ERT)
Hyperstat, Evista and, 83
Hyperthyroidism, 18

Ibuprofen, Evista and, 82
Indomethacin, Evista and, 82
Internet, 176–77

Kava, 99
anxiety and, 104
Korean ginseng, 90
fatigue and, 100
hot flashes and, 93–94
vaginal dryness and, 103

Low density lipoprotein (LDL)
  estrogen replacement therapy (ERT) affect on, 116–17
  Evista's affect on, 150–51
Lupron, 18

Mammograms, 160–61
Mayo Health Oasis, 184
Medications
  falls caused by, 49–50
  over-the-counter, 74
MEDLINE, 184
Memory loss
  Alzheimer's disease, *see* Alzheimer's disease
  estrogen and, 106
  Ginkgo biloba and, 106
  hawthorn and, 106
Menopause
  bone density loss, 30–31
  books on, 191–95
  calcium, absorption of, 12
  hot flashes, *see* Hot flashes
  night sweats, *see* Night sweats
  osteoporosis and, 110
  perimenopause, 29
  premature, 16
  smoking and, 25
  symptoms, 29–30
  urinary tract infections, 30, 100–1
  vitamin D and, 12
Menopause News, 185
Menopause Online, 185
Miacalcin, 40, 110, 111, 126
Moodiness, 103
  alternative therapies for, 104

NAMS, *see* North American Menopause Society (NAMS)
Naproxen, Evista and, 82
National Center for Homeopathy (NCH), 190
National Health Information Center (NHIC), 185
National Institute of Arthritis and Musculoskeletal and Skin Diseases (NIAMS), 186
National Institute on Aging (NIA), 186
National Osteoporosis Foundation (NOF), 187
National Women's Health Resource Center (NWHRC), 187
NCH, *see* National Center for Homeopathy (NCH)
NHIC, *see* National Health Information Center (NHIC)
NHWRC, *see* National Women's Health Resource Center (NWHRC)
NIA, *see* National Institute on Aging (NIA)
NIAMS, *see* National Institute of Arthritis and Musculoskeletal and Skin Diseases (NIAMS)
Night sweats, 30, 96–99
  estrogen replacement therapy (ERT) and, 68
NOF, *see* National Osteoporosis Foundation (NOF)
Nolvadex, 61–62, 123
Nonsteroidal anti-inflammatory drugs (NSAIDs), Evista and, 82
North American Menopause Society (NAMS), 187

Omnipen, Evista and, 82
Osteoblasts, 17, 22, 130
  growth factors and, 126
Osteoclasts, 6–7, 26, 131
  alendronate and, 124
Osteopenia, 37
Osteoporosis
  alcoholism and, 16–17, 25
  books on, 191–95
  caffeine and, *see* Caffeine

calcium supplements, *see* Calcium
compression fractures, 13
consequences of, 13
defined, 4
estrogen replacement therapy (ERT), *see* Estrogen replacement therapy (ERT)
Evista, effectiveness of, 120
exercise, *see* Exercise
facts and myths, 3
genetic role in, 15, 26
hip fractures, 13
hormone replacement therapy (HRT), *see* Estrogen replacement therapy (ERT)
informational sources, 176–77
medications available for postmenopausal women, 39–40
Osteoporosis Risk Quiz, 32, 170
physician, choosing a, 169–71
postmenopausal, 5
postmenopausal women, medications available for, 39–40
preventable condition, as, 3
prevention methods, 22–40
primary, 5
risk factors for, 14–19
risk quiz, 32, 170
secondary, 5, 18
senile, 5
smoking and, *see* Smoking
soy and, 142
statistics, 2, 3–4
support group, 170
type 1, 5
type 2, 5
types of, 5
vitamin D supplements, 23
weight-bearing exercise and, 24–25
Ovarian cancer, Evista and, 66–67

Panwarfin
Alzheimer's disease and, 108
Evista and, 82
Parathyroid hormone (PTH), 12, 127
Patients Bill of Rights, 173–74
Peak bone density, 14
Perimenopause, 29
Phytoestrogens, soy and, 142
PMS, *see* Premenstrual syndrome (PMS)
Polycillin, Evista and, 82
Postmenopausal osteoporosis, 5
Premarin, 113
Premenstrual syndrome (PMS), 30
Prevalite, Evista and, 82
Primary osteoporosis, 5
Progesterone, 38, 114
Proglycem, Evista and, 83
Prozac, 104
PTH, *see* Parathyroid hormone (PTH)

Questran Lite, Evista and, 82
Questran, Evista and, 82

Raloxifene, *see* Evista

Sahara Clinical Bone Sonometer, 34, 35, 36
Secondary osteoporosis, 5, 18
Selective estrogen receptor modulators (SERMs), 39, 60
future of, 146–47
list of available, 126–27
Senile osteoporosis, 5
SERM, *see* Selective estrogen receptor modulator (SERM)
Sexuality Information and Educational Council of the United States (SIECUS), 188
SIECUS, *see* Sexuality Information and Educational Council of the United States (SIECUS)

Single photon absorptiometry (SPA), 34, 36
Sleep hygiene, 97–99
Sleeping difficulties, 97–99
  alcohol and, 98
  alternative therapies for, 99
  caffeine and, 98
  exercise and, 98
  medications for, 99
Smoking
  Evista and, 78, 80
  heart disease and, 156
  menopause, early, 25
  osteoporosis and, 14, 17, 25
Sodium, 136
Sodium fluoride, 127
Sofarin
  Alzheimer's disease and, 108
  Evista and, 82
Soy
  hot flashes and, 95
  osteoporosis and, 142
  phytoestrogens and, 142
SPA, *see* Single photon absorptiometry (SPA)
St. John's wort, 90
  anxiety and, 104
Support groups, 170

Tamoxifen, 123
  breast cancer and, 163–64
  side effects, 164–65
  uterine cancer and, 164
TENS, *see* Transcutaneous electric nerve stimulation (TENS)
Thiazide diuretics, 127
Trabecular bone, 6
Transcutaneous electric nerve stimulation (TENS), 41–42

U.S. Department of Agriculture, 188
Urinary tract infections, 30, 100–1
Uterine cancer
  estrogen replacement therapy (ERT), *see* Estrogen replacement therapy (ERT)
  Evista, 79, 122–23
  tamoxifen and, 164

Vaginal dryness
  alternative therapies, 103
  estrogen replacement therapy (ERT) and, 68, 89, 102
  sexual discomfort and, 101–3
Valium, Evista and, 83
Vertebral fractures, 46–47
Vitamin D
  alcohol abuse and, *see* Alcoholism
  deficiency, 17–18, 49
  smoking and, 25
  sources of, 132
  supplements, 23, 64, 77, 111, 131, 134
Vitamin E, Alzheimer's disease and, 108

Warfarin
  Alzheimer's disease and, 108
  Evista and, 82
World Health Organization (WHO), 189
Wrist fractures, 47